# ONCOGENES AND TUMOR SUPPRESSOR GENES

**F. Macdonald**

*DNA Laboratory, Regional Genetics Service, East Birmingham Hospital, Bordesley Green East, Birmingham B9 5ST, U.K.*

**C. H. J. Ford**

*Oncology Research, Memorial University and the Newfoundland Cancer Treatment and Research Foundation, St John's, Newfoundland, Canada A1B 3V6*

βIOS
**SCIENTIFIC**
**PUBLISHERS**

© BIOS Scientific Publishers Limited, 1991

First published in the United Kingdom 1991 by
BIOS Scientific Publishers Limited,
St Thomas House, Becket Street, Oxford OX1 1SJ.

A CIP catalogue record for this book is available from the British Library.

ISBN 1 872 748 55 4

Typeset by HiTech Typesetters, Oxford, U.K.
Printed by Information Press Ltd, Oxford, U.K.

# PREFACE

Over the last few years, we have begun to understand the molecular basis of the malignant phenotype and identification of some of the genes involved has made a considerable impact in oncology. The aim of this book is to provide non-specialists in this field, including medical students, postgraduates and medical practitioners, with a readable text which both summarizes the scientific aspects of these genes and shows how they may be used to influence patient management. This book is not intended to cover the biology of these genes in great depth as there are already many excellent texts available, but merely to provide the reader with sufficient background to understand the subsequent chapters relevant to medical practice. The first two chapters summarize our current knowledge about the genes, the third chapter describes the techniques available for their study and the fourth and fifth chapters discuss the impact these genes have had in the diagnosis and prognosis of cancers. The final chapter covers the potential of the genes and their products as targets for therapy. Key references are given at the end of each chapter as well as suggestions for further reading.

Our thanks go to Dr Alan Cockayne and Mr Dion Morton for reading the manuscript and for helpful comments, to Dr Jonathan Waters for help with the illustrations, to all our colleagues who provided us with figures, to the Series Editor Dr Andrew Read, and BIOS Scientific Publishers Ltd for their help.

# CONTENTS

# ABBREVIATIONS

| | |
|---|---|
| ALL | acute lymphocytic leukemia |
| AML | acute myeloid leukemia |
| *APC* | adenomatous polyposis coli |
| *BCR* | breakpoint cluster region |
| BWS | Beckwith–Wiedemann Syndrome |
| CDRs | complementarity determining regions |
| CHRPE | congenital hypertrophy of retinal pigment epithelium |
| CML | chronic myeloid leukemia |
| *CSF-1* | colony-stimulating factor 1 |
| CT | computerized tomography |
| DAPI | 4,6-diamidino-2-phenylindole |
| *DCC* | deleted in colorectal cancer |
| DMs | double-minute chromosomes |
| EGF | epidermal growth factor |
| EGFR | epidermal growth factor receptor |
| FACS | fluorescence-activated cell sorter |
| FAP | familial adenomatous polyposis |
| GAP | GTPase activating protein |
| GDP | guanosine diphosphate |
| GTP | guanosine triphosphate |
| HAMA | human anti-mouse antibodies |
| HPV | human papilloma virus |
| HSRs | homogeneous-staining regions |
| LOH | loss of heterozygosity |
| *MCR* | major cluster region |
| MDS | myelodysplastic syndrome |
| MEN | multiple endocrine neoplasia |
| NF1 | Von Recklinghausen neurofibromatosis/neurofibromatosis 1 |
| NF2 | bilateral acoustic neurofibromatosis/neurofibromatosis 2 |
| N-SCLC | non-small-cell lung cancer |
| PCR | polymerase chain reaction |
| PDGF | platelet-derived growth factor |
| RB | retinoblastoma |
| RFLPs | restriction fragment-length polymorphisms |
| SCLC | small cell lung cancer |
| TGF-$\alpha$/$\beta$ | transforming growth factor $\alpha$/$\beta$ |
| VNTRs | variable number of tandem repeats |

# 1
# ONCOGENES

## 1.1 Introduction

It has been realized for many years that cancer has a genetic component. In 1914, Boveri suggested that an aberration in the genome might be responsible for the origins of cancer. This was subsequently supported by the evidence that (a) cancer, or the risk of cancer, could be inherited, (b) that mutagens could cause tumors in both animals and humans, and (c) that tumors are monoclonal in origin, that is, the cells of a tumor all show the genetic characteristics of the original transformed cell. It is only in recent years that the involvement of specific genes has been demonstrated at the molecular level.

Analysis of the development of the transformed phenotype has enabled three broad classes of genes involved in the transition from a normal cell to a malignant one to be defined. The first of these are the oncogenes – genes related to normal cellular genes whose aberrant expression contributes to malignancy. The second class of genes is the tumor suppressor genes which normally act to control cell proliferation and whose loss or inactivation is again associated with tumorigenesis. Thirdly, there is a group of genes involved in DNA repair which, when mutated, predispose the patient to developing cancer. This failure of DNA repair is seen in xeroderma pigmentosum, ataxia telangectasia, Fanconi's anemia and Bloom's Syndrome [1]. In addition, many other genes encoding proteins, such as proteinases or other enzymes capable of disrupting tissues, and vascular permeability factors have been shown to be involved in carcinogenesis. Epigenetic events such as alterations in the degree of methylation of DNA have also been detected in tumors [2].

Any combination of these changes may be found in an individual tumor. The overall progression to malignancy is therefore a complex event. Only two groups of genes, the oncogenes and the tumor suppressor genes, are discussed in this book to demonstrate how this area of research has contributed to our understanding of the tumor cell and how these genes might alter our current methods of diagnosis and treatment.

## 1.2 The multistage nature of cancer development

In 1949, Berenblum and Shublik stated from their experiments that 'the recognition that carcinogenesis is at least a two stage process should invariably

**1**

be borne in mind' [3]. Armitage and Doll took this observation a step further; in 1954, they published age/incidence curves for 17 common types of cancer. From their figures they concluded that carcinogenesis was at least a six or seven stage process [4]. Although each of these steps cannot usually be clearly defined in an individual tumor, it is clear today that there is without doubt a multistage progression to malignancy.

Tumors tend to acquire more aggressive characteristics as they develop, and in 1957 Foulds pointed out that tumor progression occurred in a stepwise fashion, each step determined by the activation, mutation or loss of specific genes [5]. Over the next two decades biochemical and cytogenetic studies demonstrated the sequential appearance of subpopulations of cells within a tumor, attributable, in part at least, to changes in the genes themselves.

Evidence suggests that in the majority of cases cancers arise from a single cell which has acquired some heritable form of growth advantage [6]. This initiation step is believed frequently to be caused by some form of genotoxic agent such as radiation or a chemical carcinogen. The cells at this stage, although altered at the DNA level, are phenotypically normal. Further mutational events involving genes responsible for control of cell growth lead to the emergence of clones with additional properties associated with tumor cell progression. Finally, additional changes allow the outgrowth of clones with metastatic potential. Each of these successive events is likely to make the cell more unstable so that the risk of subsequent changes increases. Animal models of carcinogenesis, primarily based on models of skin cancer development in mice, have enabled these steps to be divided into initiation events, promotion, malignant transformation and metastasis [6] (*Figure 1.1*).

Each of these sequential changes may result from a variety of different mechanisms. One such mechanism is a mutation in a normal cellular gene controlling cell growth and proliferation,which confers on the cell some potential for malignant transformation. The mutation converts a normal cellular gene into an oncogene.

## 1.3 Viruses and cancer

For almost 30 years, it has been known that DNA viruses such as SV40 virus and RNA viruses such as the retrovirus, Rous sarcoma virus, are capable of transforming those cells they infect. These viruses are associated primarily with animals and rarely cause human disease, although a few examples are known (*Table 1.1*). The viruses are particularly important because they have taught us a great deal about the molecular basis for transformation and have led to the identification of cellular oncogenes.

Most of this information has come from studies of the retroviruses. These RNA viruses encode three genes, *gag, pol* and *env* which produce a core protein, a reverse transcriptase and envelope glycoproteins, respectively (*Figure 1.2*). In those viruses capable of causing malignant transformation, a fourth gene, the oncogene, has been found.

A clue as to how these genes might be involved in the pathogenesis of cancers came in 1976 when a group studying the Rous sarcoma virus, which

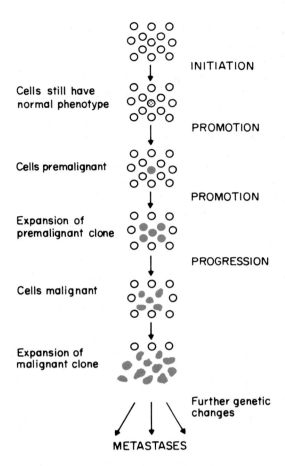

INITIATION

Cells still have
normal phenotype

PROMOTION

Cells premalignant

PROMOTION

Expansion of
premalignant clone

PROGRESSION

Cells malignant

Expansion of
malignant clone

Further genetic
changes

METASTASES

**Figure 1.1:** *Multistage
progression to malignancy.*

**Table 1.1:** *Viruses associated with human cancers*

| Virus | Associated tumors |
|---|---|
| DNA viruses | |
|   Epstein–Barr | Burkitt's lymphoma |
| | Nasopharyngeal cancer |
|   Hepatitis B | Liver cancer |
|   Papilloma virus | Benign warts |
| | Cervical cancer |
| RNA viruses | |
|   Human immunodeficiency virus (HIV-1) | Kaposi's sarcoma |
|   Human T-cell leukemia virus Type I | |
|     (HTLV-1) | Adult T-cell leukemia |
|   HTLV-2 | Hairy cell leukemia |
|   HTLV-5 | Cutaneous T-cell leukemia |

Retroviral genome

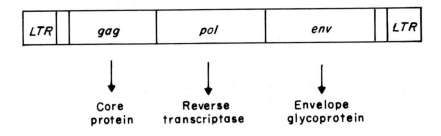

Oncogenic retrovirus

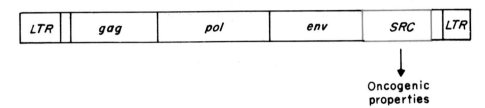

**Figure 1.2:** *The retroviral genome.*

causes malignancy in chickens, showed that the *SRC* oncogene carried by the virus was not viral in origin but had been picked up by the virus from the host genome, a process termed transduction [7]. This was possible because the retrovirus uses its reverse transcriptase enzyme to make a DNA copy of its genome. The DNA copy can integrate reversibly into the host genome (*Figure 1.3*). By recombination between viral and host DNA, the retroviruses 'kidnap' a host gene which then becomes part of the viral genome. The resulting virus is usually defective at replication, but can transform host cells following re-infection.

Using DNA probes specific for the oncogene carried by the retroviruses, further homologous genes were identified in the normal vertebrate genome (*Table 1.2*) and named after the virus in which they were first identified (*v-onc*). These genes are activated when transduced by the retrovirus either because the gene is altered, resulting in a protein with abnormal activity, or because the gene is brought under the control of a viral promoter, leading to aberrant expression. With reference to their potential function in tumor development, the original cellular genes were termed proto-oncogenes.

Retroviruses can also activate proto-oncogenes more directly by a process known as insertional mutagenesis. In this process, the insertion of a DNA copy of the retrovirus into the cellular genome close to a proto-oncogene is sufficient to cause abnormal activation of that gene. This has been demonstrated for the *INT1* gene which is activated in breast cancer in mice

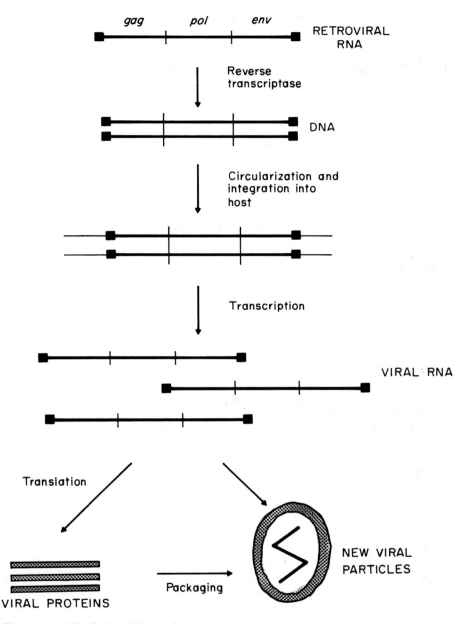

**Figure 1.3**: *Life cycle of the retrovirus.*

infected with the mouse mammary tumor virus. Most of the proto-oncogenes identified in this way are identical to those already found via transforming retroviruses, although a few additional genes such as *EV1I* have also been found.

As few retroviruses had been shown to be the cause of human cancers, it was still not clear how these genes associated with the retroviruses might relate to the pathogenesis of cancer in man. It was only when it was shown that human tumors contained activated oncogenes homologous to those found in the retroviruses, but with no viral intermediary, that this whole area of research expanded rapidly.

**Table 1.2:** *Retroviral oncogenes*

| Oncogene | Virus | Tumor |
|---|---|---|
| *v-abl* | Abelson leukemia virus | Leukemia |
| *v-erb A* | Avian erythroblastosis virus | Helps *v-erb B* |
| *v-erb B* | Avian erythroblastosis virus | Erythroleukemia |
| *v-fms* | Feline sarcoma virus | Sarcoma |
| *v-H-ras* | Rat sarcoma virus (Harvey strain) | Sarcoma |
| *v-K-ras* | Rat sarcoma virus (Kirsten strain) | Sarcoma |
| *v-jun* | Avian sarcoma virus | Fibrosarcoma |
| *v-myb* | Avian myeloblastosis virus | Myeloblastosis |
| *v-myc* | Avian myelocytomatosis virus | Leukemia |
| *v-sis* | Simian sarcoma virus | Sarcoma |
| *v-src* | Rous sarcoma virus | Sarcoma |

## 1.4 Cellular oncogenes

Whilst research into the retroviral oncogenes continued, more direct methods of identifying oncogenic sequences in the human genome were examined. A DNA transfection assay was used as a method of identifying those sequences in tumor cells which were responsible for uncontrolled cell proliferation. DNA was extracted from human tumors and sheared into fragments. These were then transfected into a mouse-derived cell line called NIH-3T3 so that random fragments were incorporated into its genome. As a result, some cells were transformed and could be identified by their loss of contact inhibition which caused cells to pile up *in vitro* (*Figure 1.4*). These transformed cells were also capable of producing tumors when injected into athymic (nude) mice. The genome of the transformed cells was analyzed and shown to contain an oncogene which in many cases was similar to one which had been identified in the retroviruses [8] (*Table 1.3*). This transfection assay did not give a positive result with all tumors. Only about 20% of tumors contained oncogenes which could be identified in this way and about one-quarter of these belonged to the *RAS* gene family. Additional oncogenes were identified by alternative strategies.

It had long been known that some tumors carry a consistent chromosome translocation. In the case of chronic myeloid leukemia (CML), this is a reciprocal translocation between chromosomes 9 and 22 (see Section 1.4.2). In

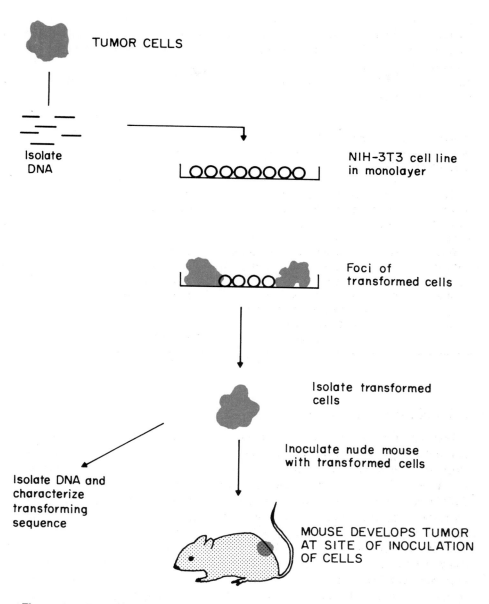

**Figure 1.4:** *DNA transfection assay.*

Burkitt's lymphoma, there is a reciprocal translocation between chromosome 8 and, in the majority of cases, chromosome 14, although either chromosome 2 or chromosome 22 is occasionally involved. In both examples the breakpoints were shown to coincide with the location of oncogenes already identified from retroviral studies – *ABL* on chromosome 9 and *MYC* on chromosome 8. Other translocations in tumors identified the sites of further oncogenes (*Table 1.3*). In a comprehensive study of 5345 tumors [9], the distribution of cancer-specific breakpoints was compared with the site of 26 cellular oncogenes. Nineteen of the 26 oncogenes were located at cancer-associated chromosome breakpoints.

Two other chromosome abnormalities observed in tumors have also identified the location of oncogenes (*Table 1.3*). Both the development of homogeneous-staining regions (HSRs) and formation of double-minute chromosomes (DMs; *Figure 1.5*) were associated with oncogene amplification. Some oncogenes identified in this way, for example, *MYC*, had previously been detected by other techniques, but other genes such as *MYCN*, associated with neuroblastomas, and *MYCL*, found in small cell lung carcinomas, were first revealed in this way [10].

**Table 1.3**: *Methods of oncogene identification in human tumors*

| Method of identification | Oncogene |
| --- | --- |
| Amplification | *ERBB2, MYCL, MYCN* |
| Chromosomal translocation | *ABL, BCL1, BCL2, MYC* |
| Homology to retroviruses | *HRAS, KRAS, SRC* |
| Insertional mutagenesis | *EVI1, INT1* |
| Transfection assay | *MAS, MET, MYC, RAS, TRK* |

Currently about 60 different oncogenes have been identified, which have arisen through alterations to a normal cellular gene (see Appendix A for the location of some of these). The repeated identification of the same oncogenes by means of different techniques from different sources, as well as in the retroviruses, suggests that although some genes are as yet undiscovered, the majority have now been found.

The importance of these genes to the cell is clear as there is sequence conservation from organisms such as yeast, through the invertebrates and vertebrates to man. In the normal cell, the expression of these proto-oncogenes is tightly controlled and they are transcribed at the appropriate stages of growth and development of cells. However, alterations in these genes or their control sequences leads to inappropriate expression. What therefore are the functions of these genes and how are they converted into genes capable of contributing to malignant progression?

### 1.4.1 Function of the proto-oncogenes

Subsequent work has supported the prediction that the proto-oncogenes would be involved in the basic essential functions of the cell related to control of cell growth and differentiation. The products of these genes are detected at many different cellular locations as shown in *Figure 1.6*. Their roles in the cell

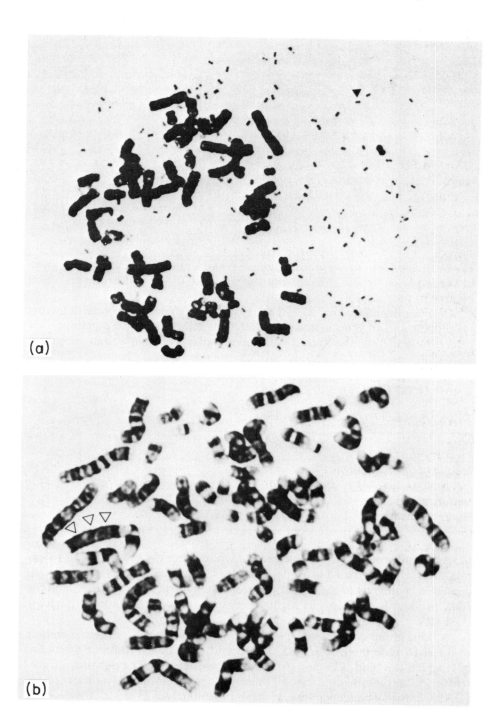

**Figure 1.5:** *Examples of (a) DMs and (b) HSRs (arrowed). Figure courtesy of Dr J. Waters, Regional Cytogenetics Laboratory, East Birmingham Hospital, U.K.*

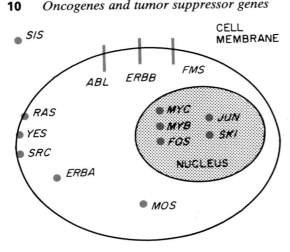

**Figure 1.6:** *Cellular locations of oncogene products.*

can be divided into four groups (*Table 1.4*) and a mutation in any one of these genes might be expected to disrupt the response of the cell to signals which control its growth [11].

Cells are capable of producing and responding to their own growth factors – a process known as autocrine secretion. This is thought to play an important role in stimulating the growth of tumor cells. The first group of proto-oncogenes are therefore those which encode growth factors. The *SIS* oncogene codes for a protein homologous to a subunit of platelet-derived growth factor (PDGF).

**Table 1.4:** *Role of proto-oncogenes in the cell*

| Role | Oncogene | Homology |
|------|----------|----------|
| Growth factor | SIS | PDGF |
| Growth factor receptors | ERBB, FMS | EGFR, CSF1R |
| Nuclear oncogenes | JUN, MYB, MYC | |
| Signal transducers | ABL, MOS, RAF, RAS, SRC | |

A second group of proto-oncogenes encode either the growth factor receptors themselves or their functional homologs. Thus the product of the *ERBB* gene is homologous to the epidermal growth factor receptor (EGFR) and the *FMS* product is homologous to the receptor for colony-stimulating factor 1 (CSF1R).

A third group comprises the signal transducers. The three main members of the *RAS* gene family—*HRAS*, *KRAS* and *NRAS* each code for a protein, p21, which can bind GTP and exhibits GTPase activity. The normal p21 protein also interacts with a cytoplasmic protein, GTPase activating protein, (GAP), which speeds up the transition from *RAS*–GTP to *RAS*–GDP. Although the exact mode of action of p21 is still not completely clear, it appears that *RAS*–p21 mediates changes in intracellular metabolism in response to signals from the cell surface receptors (*Figure 1.7*). Other proteins

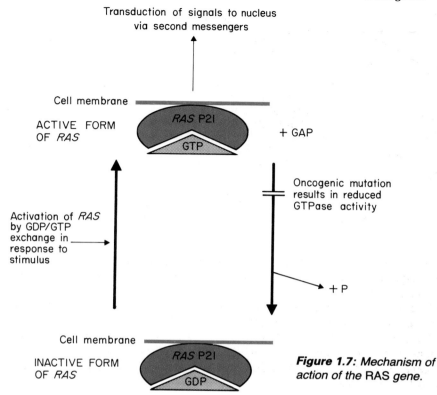

Transduction of signals to nucleus
via second messengers

Cell membrane

ACTIVE FORM
OF *RAS*

RAS P21

GTP

+ GAP

Oncogenic mutation
results in reduced
GTPase activity

Activation of *RAS*
by GDP/GTP
exchange in
response to
stimulus

+ P

Cell membrane

INACTIVE FORM
OF *RAS*

RAS P21

GDP

**Figure 1.7:** *Mechanism of action of the* RAS *gene.*

such as the G-protein in the adenylate cyclase system show homology to p21 in the GTP binding domain [12].

The signals for stimulation of growth from the growth factors and their receptors must ultimately act, via a number of second messengers, at the level of gene expression. Second messengers are essentially signal transducers and transmitters which function by activating a protein cascade. This is controlled at the level of protein phosphorylation by the protein kinases. Products of several of the membrane-associated proto-oncogenes such as *SRC* and *ABL* have tyrosine kinase activity, as do several of those which act in the cytoplasm, such as the products of *RAF1* and *MOS*. In addition, several transmembrane growth factor receptors have protein kinase activity associated with the cytoplasmic domain.

The final group of proto-oncogenes are those involved in the control of gene expression by their action on DNA itself. This is the final site of action for messages sent from the growth factors and is the level at which control of growth and proliferation ultimately operates. Several of the proto-oncogene proteins have been shown to bind to and presumably control the transcription of genes, for example, *MYC*, *FOS* and *JUN*. The *MYC* gene product, p62, is believed to be essential for cell proliferation and differentiation. Expression of *MYC* is linked to entry and exit from the cell cycle and p62 has been postulated to play a role in DNA replication, possibly binding those regions which serve as initiation sites for DNA synthesis [13]. The product of *JUN* is known to be a

**Table 1.5:** *Mechanisms of oncogene activation*

| Method of activation | Oncogene |
| --- | --- |
| Amplification | *ERBB2, MYB, MYC* |
| Loss of control mechanism | |
|     Insertional mutagenesis | *INT1, INT2* |
|     Translocation | *MYC* |
| Structural alteration | *ABL, HRAS, KRAS, SRC* |

transcription factor. These are factors which are thought to form the initiation complex from which RNA polymerase starts. Mutations in these genes will therefore alter transcription rates.

The various mechanisms by which the proto-oncogenes are activated to produce a gene with oncogenic potential are described in the next section.

### 1.4.2 Mechanisms of oncogene activation

*Table 1.5* shows the three main ways by which proto-oncogenes are activated. The first mechanism is production of an abnormal product which can occur in at least three different ways. Point mutations have been described in several oncogenes but have been studied most extensively in genes of the *RAS* family. Amino acid substitutions have been detected, particularly at positions 12, 13 and 61, in a variety of tumors including breast, lung and colon. Activation of the protein to an oncogenic form is also possible at positions 56, 63, 116 and 119, but these changes have not been seen in human tumors. These substitutions all alter the structure of the normal protein resulting in abnormal activity. Oncogenic forms of *RAS* produce a protein with decreased GTPase activity which prevents deactivation of the *RAS*–GTP complex, leading to prolonged stimulation of signals from the growth factor receptors [12].

Another oncogenic mutation of proto-oncogenes results in truncation of the protein as seen in *v-src* where part of the C-terminus of the protein is absent. This results in a protein with increased tyrosine kinase activity.

Finally, abnormal products of the oncogenes are detected following chromosomal translocation, resulting in the production of a fusion protein. An example of this is seen in CML where chromosome 9 is translocated to chromosome 22. This places the *ABL* oncogene on chromosome 9 next to the breakpoint cluster region (*BCR*) of the Philadelphia gene on chromosome 22 (*Figure 1.8* and Section 4.6.4). A fusion gene is formed which in turn produces an abnormal fusion protein. The fusion protein shows abnormal tyrosine kinase activity which accounts for its transforming ability.

The second mechanism of activation is over-production of the normal protein by amplification of the proto-oncogene [10]. For example, amplification of the *MYC* gene is found in some breast and colorectal cancers. Amplification of the *MYCN* gene is consistently associated with late-stage neuroblastomas. In breast cancer, amplification of the *ERBB2* gene is a common finding. The *RAS* oncogene, which is frequently activated by point mutation, has also been found to be amplified in certain human tumors.

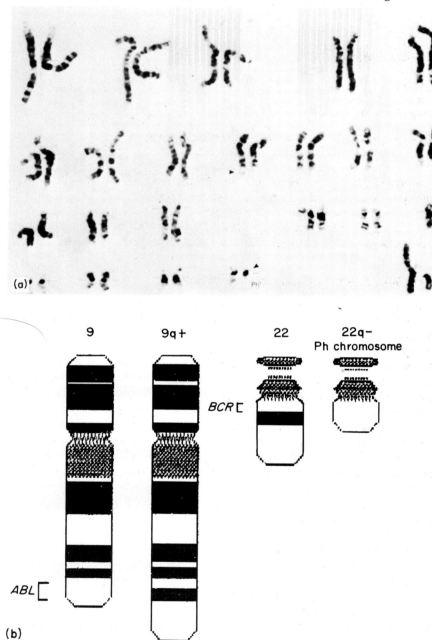

**Figure 1.8:** *(a) Karyotype from a case of CML showing the Ph¹ chromosome (arrowed on bottom row) and (b) ideogram of the t(9;22). Figure courtesy of Dr P. Fisher, Cytogenetics Laboratory, Department of Haematological Medicine, Addenbrookes Hospital, Cambridge, U.K.*

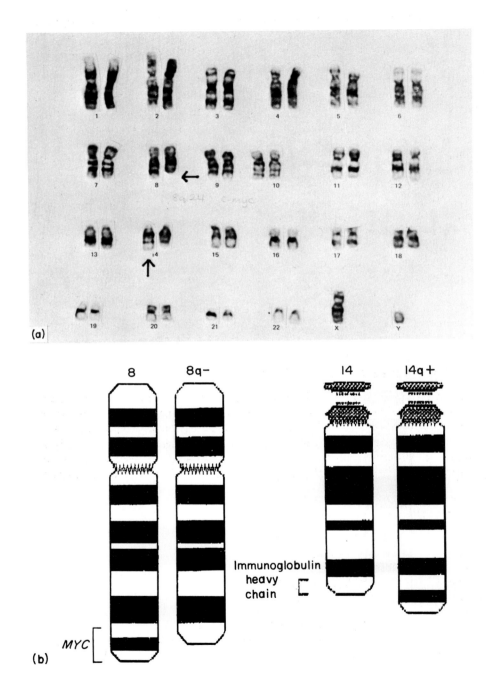

**Figure 1.9**: *(a) Karyotype from a Burkitt's lymphoma containing a t(8;14) and (b) ideogram of the translocation. Figure courtesy of the Regional Cytogenetics Laboratory, East Birmingham Hospital, U.K.*

The third mechanism of activation occurs through loss of appropriate control mechanisms. This has been described in an earlier section for the retroviral oncogenes, where insertional mutagenesis causes transcriptional activation. Cellular oncogenes also show loss of normal transcription control through chromosomal translocation typified by the 8;14 translocation seen in Burkitt's lymphoma [14] (*Figure 1.9*). Following the juxtaposition of the *MYC* oncogene on chromosome 8 to the *IGH* gene locus on chromosome 14, there is constitutive expression of the transposed *MYC* gene, that is, the normal control of the *MYC* gene is overridden by the control mechanisms of the *IGH* gene. As with amplification of the proto-oncogenes, the effect of this mechanism is the over-production of the gene product.

There is no single consistent mechanism of activation of any one oncogene. Thus *RAS* is primarily activated by point mutation but amplification is also found, *MYC* is amplified in many tumors but abnormal expression is also associated with deregulation following chromosomal translocation. Whatever the mechanism for the activation of these genes, the end result is to produce a protein which can cause abnormal growth.

Although the main area of research is in how these genes relate to the development of tumors, abnormal products of the proto-oncogenes are also associated with non-malignant conditions such as arthritis, proliferative vasculitis and also in the process of wound healing where proliferation or differentiation are either required or found to be disordered.

## 1.5 Oncogenes in human tumors

In most groups of tumors so far examined for the presence of an oncogene, such a gene has been found. A few of the most common tumors and associated oncogenes are shown in *Table 1.6* but the list is far from complete. The value of these oncogenes as diagnostic or prognostic markers is discussed fully in Chapter 4. In many tumors such as Burkitt's lymphoma or CML, the presence of the oncogene is likely to have an important, although not necessarily

**Table 1.6**: Oncogenes in human tumors

| Tumor | Associated oncogene |
|---|---|
| Bladder | HRAS, KRAS |
| Brain | ERBB1, SIS |
| Breast | ERBB2, HRAS, MYC |
| Cervical | MYC |
| Colorectal | HRAS, KRAS, MYB, MYC |
| Gastric | ERBB1, HST, MYB, MYC, NRAS, YES |
| Lung | ERBB1, HRAS, KRAS, MYC, MYCL, MYCN |
| Melanoma | HRAS |
| Neuroblastoma | MYCN |
| Ovarian | ERBB2, KRAS |
| Pancreas | KRAS, MYC |
| Prostate | MYC |
| Testicular | MYC |

primary, role in the development of the tumor. In other tumors it is not clear exactly what role the presence of the oncogene has to play in the development of the cancer. Some oncogenes are likely to be detected not because they have been specifically activated, but because control of normal cell growth has been disrupted, leading to their subsequent activation. For example, in tumors formed following inoculation of mice with a fibroblast cell line previously transfected with human *MYC* or mutated *HRAS*, elevated levels of the transfected gene could be detected, but there was also elevated expression of the endogenous *ABL* and *FOS* genes. This result suggests that one gene might be able to destabilize the cell sufficiently to provide an environment in which further changes in other oncogenes are likely [15].

Here we need to return to the concept of cancer as a phenotype which arises following a number of sequential alterations in the cell. We stated earlier that a single mutational event was not enough for a tumor to develop, but we have described examples of oncogenes which act in a dominant manner and which in some cases have been detected only by their ability to transform the NIH-3T3 cell line. This experiment needs to be seen in perspective. The NIH-3T3 cell line is not normal but has undergone a number of mutational events during its establishment in culture. Insertion of a single oncogene into a totally normal cell line will not cause it to transform without considerable manipulation of its expression. Much evidence now suggests that there is collaboration between different oncogenes and that this is necessary to produce the fully transformed phenotype.

In model systems it was initially demonstrated that whereas a single oncogene was insufficient for transformation, collaboration between genes such as *RAS* and *MYC* or *RAS* and *p53* could result in full transformation. Some of the observations have been demonstrated more directly in transgenic mice. In this model, a fragment of DNA containing an oncogene linked to a suitable promoter can be injected into a fertilized mouse egg. Often this recombinant fragment of DNA is integrated into the mouse genome and may be expressed in many tissues or only a few depending on the tissue specificity of the promoter. When this was tried with either *MYC* or *RAS* alone, few of the progeny produced tumors, although the introduced gene was generally expressed. Only the occasional cell which had undergone further changes became transformed. Not all the progeny from a cross between two transgenic mice, one carrying *MYC* and the other *RAS*, developed tumors, although an increase in the number of tumors was seen compared with either parent [16].

This interaction between the oncogenes is only one of the processes involved in malignant development. We now know that a further group of genes, which act in a growth-regulatory rather than a growth-promoting fashion, are also involved with each other and with the oncogenes – these genes are the subject of the next chapter.

## References

1. Cleaver, J.E. and Karentz, A. (1987) *BioEssays,* **6,** 122.
2. Goelz, S., Vogelstein, B., Hamilton, S.R. and Feinberg, A.P. (1985) *Science,* **228,** 187.
3. Berenblum, I. and Shubik, P. (1949) *Br. J. Cancer,* **3,** 109.

4. Armitage, P. and Doll, R. (1949) *Br. J. Cancer,* **3,** 109.
5. Foulds, L. (1957) *Cancer Res.,* **17,** 355.
6. Nowell, P.C. (1976) *Science,* **194,** 23.
7. Stehelin, D., Varmus, H.V., Bishop, J.M. and Vogt, P.K. (1976) *Nature,* **260,** 170.
8. Shih, C., Padhy, L.C., Murray, M. and Weinberg, R.A. (1981) *Nature,* **290,** 261.
9. Heim, S. and Mitelman, F. (1987) *Hum. Genet.,* **75,** 70.
10. Schwab, M. and Amler, L.C. (1990) *Genes, Chromo. Cancer,* **1,** 181.
11. Hunter, T. (1985) *Sci. American,* **253,** 60.
12. Barbacid, M. (1987) *Ann. Rev. Biochem.,* **56,** 779.
13. Erisman, M.D. and Astrin, S.M. (1988) in *The Oncogene Handbook* (E.P. Reddy, A.M. Skalka and T. Curran, eds). Elsevier, New York, p. 341.
14. Klein, G. and Klein, E. (1985) *Immunol. Today,* **6,** 208.
15. Wyllie, A.H., Rose, K.A., Morris, R.G., Steel, C.M., Foster, E. and Spandidos, D.A. (1987) *Br. J. Cancer,* **56,** 251.
16. Sinn, E. (1987) *Cell,* **49,** 465.

## Further reading

Buick, K.B., Liu, E.T. and Larnick, J.W. (1988) *Oncogenes: an introduction to the concept of cancer genes.* Springer-Verlag, New York.

# 2
# TUMOR SUPPRESSOR GENES

A second group of genes which play an important role in tumorigenesis are the tumor suppressor genes. These are defined as genes involved in the control of abnormal growth and whose loss or inactivation is associated with the development of malignancy. The literature abounds with different names for these genes which may cause some confusion; these include ortho-genes, emerogenes, flatogenes and onco-suppressor genes. Most commonly, they are described as tumor suppressor genes or anti-oncogenes. As the genes do not always act directly on an oncogene, this latter term is a misnomer. The term tumor suppressor gene also has its limitations. As the control of growth is likely to involve a number of genetic mechanisms, it is not clear that a single gene can abrogate all of them. However, until the debate on the correct terminology reaches its conclusion this term will be used here.

Tumor suppressor genes are more difficult to identify than oncogenes. Introduction of an oncogene into an untransformed cell culture and identification of the resulting transformed colonies is relatively straightforward. It is not as easy to identify untransformed revertants on a background of transformed cells. Two different techniques have been used to establish the existence of tumor suppressor genes in man.

## 2.1 Evidence for the existence of tumor suppressor genes

The best studied examples of tumor suppressor genes are found in the fruit fly, *Drosophila melanogaster*. Over 25 different genes which cause tumors by homozygous recessive mutations have been identified. Some of these have been cloned and one – lethal(2)giant larvae – shows suppression of tumor formation when re-introduced into the germ-line.

Evidence from two types of study supports the existence of tumor suppressor genes in man. These are (a) the suppression of malignancy in somatic cell hybrids and (b) a consistent loss of chromosomal regions, initially seen in hereditary cancers and subsequently also shown in sporadic cancers.

### 2.1.1 Suppression of malignancy by cell fusion

The earliest evidence for tumor suppressor genes pre-dates the discovery of oncogenes by over 20 years. Harris and colleagues showed that when malignant

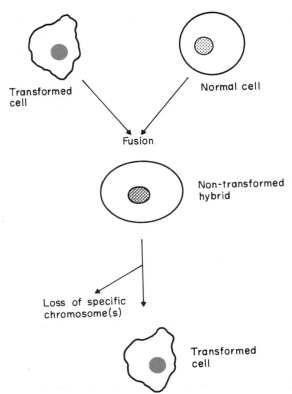

**Figure 2.1**: *Production of somatic cell hybrids.*

cells were fused with normal diploid cells, the resulting hybrids were non-tumorigenic as determined by their inability to grow in immunocompromised hosts [1] (*Figure 2.1*). This suppression of malignancy was dependent on retention of a specific chromosome. As the hybrids were unstable, there was random loss of chromosomes and when a particular chromosome was lost, malignant clones were once again capable of growth *in vivo*. The assumption was that the chromosome which was lost contained the tumor suppressor gene(s). Fusion of two malignant cells also gave rise to non-tumorigenic hybrids suggesting complementation between lesions. Detailed cytogenetic analyses of the hybrids have identified specific chromosomes involved in the suppression of the malignant phenotype. For example, the presence of chromosome 11 from the normal partner is necessary to maintain the suppression of the malignant phenotype when HeLa cervical carcinoma cells are fused with normal fibroblasts. This result was confirmed by introducing a single fibroblast chromosome 11 into HeLa cells by microcell fusion; the malignant phenotype of the cervical cancer cells was suppressed [2].

Although tumorigenesis is suppressed in hybrids between HeLa cells and normal fibroblasts, the hybrids still behave as transformed cells *in vitro*. This suggests that transformation and tumorigenicity are under separate genetic controls. Other characteristics of tumor cells, such as immortalization and metastatic ability, can also be suppressed in hybrids suggesting that a number of different genes are involved in the tumorigenic phenotype [2].

Reversion of the malignant phenotype can also be demonstrated in the presence of an activated oncogene. Non-tumorigenic hybrids have been produced following fusion of cell lines carrying either activated *NRAS* or *HRAS* genes with normal fibroblasts. These phenotypically normal hybrids, and also tumorigenic revertants, still express the product of the respective oncogene [2].

### 2.1.2 Tumor suppressor genes in hereditary cancers – the retinoblastoma model

A second piece of evidence for the existence of tumor suppressor genes came from studies of hereditary cancers. These are cancers where there is a clear pattern of inheritance – usually autosomal dominant – with a tendency for earlier age of onset than for sporadic tumors.

The prototype for studies on hereditary cancers is retinoblastoma, a childhood cancer which occurs in two forms and affects the retina (*Figure 2.2*). Forty per cent of cases are hereditary and tumors frequently arise in both eyes. The remaining 60% of cases are sporadic and characteristically tumors are seen in only one eye. In 1971, from studies of age/incidence curves, Knudson

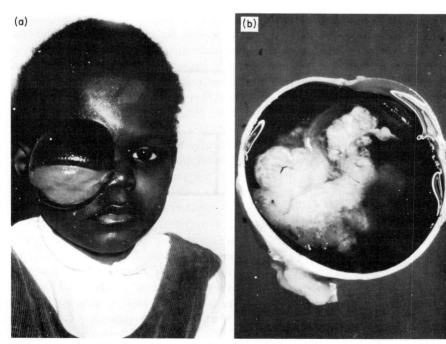

**Figure 2.2:** (a) Retinoblastoma and (b) histology from the same tumor. Figure courtesy of MRC Clinical Oncology and Therapeutic Unit, Cambridge, U.K.

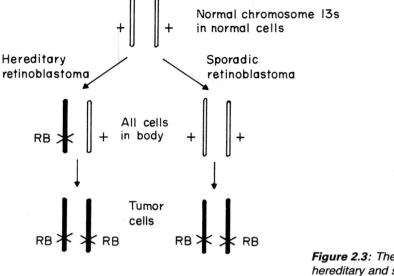

*Figure 2.3: The origin of hereditary and sporadic retinoblastomas.*

[3] postulated that the disease arose from two sequential mutational events. In the hereditary form of the disease, one mutation is inherited in the germ-line and is phenotypically harmless. A second 'hit' occurring in a retinal cell causes the tumor (*Figure 2.3*). As there are a large number of retinoblasts in the eye (over $10^7$), which are all at risk because they already carry one mutation, a second 'hit' will occur frequently enough to cause a high proportion of tumors in at least one eye and often in both. In the sporadic form of the disease, both mutations occur in the somatic tissue (*Figure 2.3*). The probability of two mutations occurring in the same cell is low, therefore the disease is both rare and unilateral [3].

This 'two-hit' hypothesis has subsequently been confirmed by identification of mutations or deletions of the gene and more recently by analysis of the cloned retinoblastoma gene itself. Before such an analysis was possible, the retinoblastoma locus had to be mapped to a specific chromosome. A number of patients were identified with a cytogenetically visible deletion in the region of band q14 of chromosome 13 (*Figure 2.4*) and it was inferred that the retinoblastoma gene (*RB1*) lay in this region. Studies of the polymorphic enzyme, esterase D, which had previously been mapped to 13q14, supported the evidence for *RB1* in this area. In families with hereditary retinoblastoma, close linkage was demonstrated between esterase D alleles and retinoblastoma, suggesting that the two genes had to be close. In non-hereditary cases, approximately 20% of retinoblastomas were shown to have an abnormality; usually absence or a deletion in one copy of chromosome 13, and reduced levels of esterase D were detected in the tumor [4]. Patients with two detectable variants of esterase D in somatic tissues had only one variant

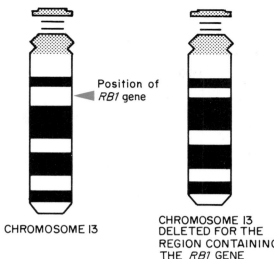

Position of *RB1* gene

CHROMOSOME 13

CHROMOSOME 13
DELETED FOR THE
REGION CONTAINING
THE *RB1* GENE

**Figure 2.4:** *Deletion of 13q14 as seen in retinoblastomas.*

present in their tumors. These studies suggested that in tumors there was loss or deletion of part of chromosome 13 and it was assumed that there was a mutation in the *RB1* gene on the remaining copy of chromosome 13 [5].

These changes were confirmed at the molecular level by Cavanee and colleagues [6] using the loss of heterozygosity test which has been widely used for the detection of tumor suppressor genes. The loss of heterozygosity test depends on differences in the lengths of DNA fragments generated by digestion of genomic DNA with restriction enzymes. These restriction fragment-length polymorphisms (RFLPs) present within the population can be detected by DNA probes specific for the DNA fragment of interest. In the case of retinoblastoma, the probes selected for use were located on 13q. Patients suitable for study were those who had different sized fragments of DNA (alleles) on each of the two chromosome 13s in their somatic tissue, that is, they were heterozygous. When tumors from the same patients were analyzed, only one of the two alleles was present (*Figure 2.5*). This loss of heterozygosity can occur by a number of possible mechanisms (*Figure 2.6*), including loss of the normal chromosome possibly followed by reduplication of the abnormal one, an interstitial deletion of the normal chromosome, or a recombination event resulting in two copies of the deficient allele. Most of the mechanisms shown in *Figure 2.6* result in loss of heterozygosity along the majority of the chromosome [6].

Narrowing the region containing the *RB1* gene made it feasible to clone the gene and study the mutations at a molecular level. Independently, three groups isolated the DNA segment which had the properties of the *RB1* gene, using basically similar approaches [7–9]. This process of identifying a gene without knowing anything about its function, product or even its location in the genome is termed 'reverse genetics' and is shown schematically in *Figure 2.7* for *RB1*. A DNA sequence (H3.8) was identified which had been shown to detect deletions in a number of retinoblastomas. Based on the assumption that

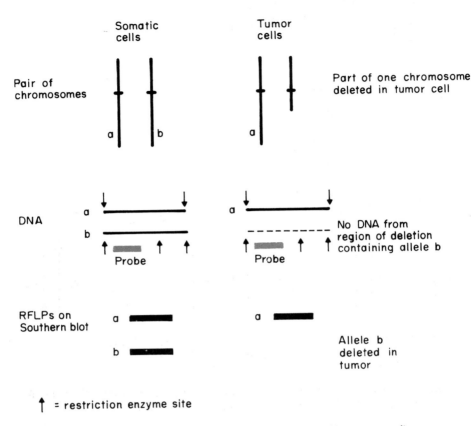

**Figure 2.5:** *RFLP analysis as a means of detecting loss of heterozygosity.*

this sequence must lie close to the *RB1* gene, a number of chromosome walks were carried out and fragments of DNA present in single copies were identified. These were used to probe DNA from humans and other species and one sequence was found to be conserved across species suggesting that it was perhaps a coding exon of a gene. Hybridization of this sequence to RNA from retinal cell lines showed that it recognized a 4.7 kb mRNA. Finally, the conserved sequence was used to isolate a cDNA clone encoding the *RB1* gene. There were several lines of evidence which verified that this was the correct sequence: (a) structural aberrations, including deletions, were seen in some retinoblastomas and osteosarcomas, (b) absence or abnormal expression of the RNA transcript was detected in tumors, and (c) a structural change in the fibroblasts of a patient with bilateral disease and a second mutation in the tumor was detected, confirming Knudson's hypothesis. The native RB protein was isolated using antisera raised against a synthetic fusion protein, which had been produced by inserting part of the *RB1* cDNA into an expression vector. The RB protein has a mass of 110 kd and is a phosphoprotein with DNA-binding activity. It is absent from retinoblastoma cell lines [10]. The *RB1* gene

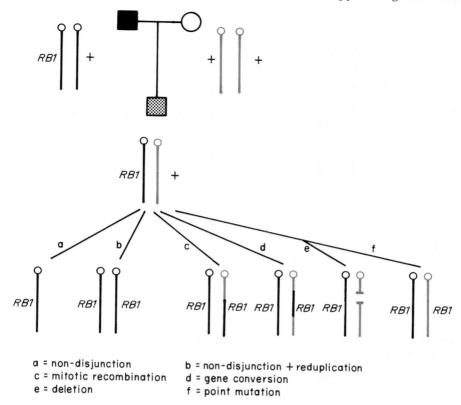

a = non-disjunction     b = non-disjunction + reduplication
c = mitotic recombination     d = gene conversion
e = deletion     f = point mutation

**Figure 2.6:** *Mechanism of loss of heterozygosity. Figure reproduced with permission from* Nature **305**, 779. *Copyright* © 1983. *Macmillan Magazines Ltd.*

is now known to span approximately 200 kb of DNA and is made up of one large exon and 26 small exons [11].

As the cDNA probe can be used to show germ-line as well as somatic mutations, it can be used to help in the diagnosis of retinoblastoma (see Chapter 5). It has also been used to identify changes in a wide range of tumors. Some of these changes, such as those seen in osteosarcomas, were expected as these tumors frequently arise in retinoblastoma patients later in life. The unexpected observation is that mutations in the *RB1* gene can be detected in unrelated tumors including breast, colon and lung. This suggests that the *RB1* gene may play an important general role in tumorigenesis.

Definitive proof that the *RB1* gene is a tumor suppressor has come from a study where the gene was introduced into retinoblastoma or osteosarcoma cell lines by means of a retroviral vector. The endogenous *RB1* gene was inactive in the cells, but expression of the exogenous *RB1* gene produced revertants which could no longer produce tumors in nude mice.

The picture for retinoblastoma is now clear and confirms Knudson's 'two hit' hypothesis. The tumor only occurs when both copies of the *RB1* gene are altered or lost. Therefore the tumor phenotype is recessive. However, the

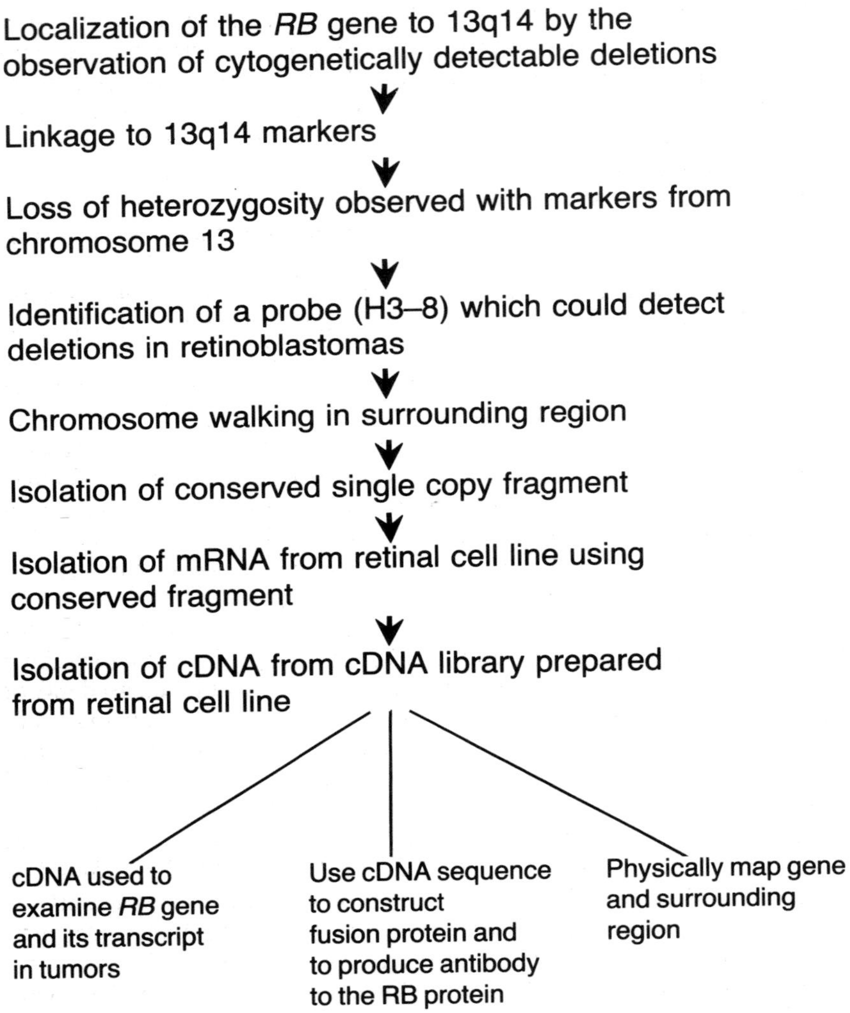

Localization of the *RB* gene to 13q14 by the observation of cytogenetically detectable deletions

▼

Linkage to 13q14 markers

▼

Loss of heterozygosity observed with markers from chromosome 13

▼

Identification of a probe (H3–8) which could detect deletions in retinoblastomas

▼

Chromosome walking in surrounding region

▼

Isolation of conserved single copy fragment

▼

Isolation of mRNA from retinal cell line using conserved fragment

▼

Isolation of cDNA from cDNA library prepared from retinal cell line

| cDNA used to examine *RB* gene and its transcript in tumors | Use cDNA sequence to construct fusion protein and to produce antibody to the RB protein | Physically map gene and surrounding region |

**Figure 2.7:** *Reverse genetics and identification of* RB1.

tumor is inherited as if it were dominantly expressed, because the likelihood of the second mutation in the retinal cells is close to 100%. This 'two hit' model has subsequently been found to be applicable to a number of other hereditary cancers discussed in the following sections.

## 2.2 Hereditary cancers

### 2.2.1 Wilms tumor

A 'two hit' mutational model has also been proposed for Wilms tumor. This is a childhood renal tumor with both a hereditary and a non-hereditary form, the former constituting only about 1% of cases [12]. Bilateral tumors occur in approximately 20% of familial cases. Wilms tumor is also associated with a complex of other conditions – aniridia, genito-urinary abnormalities and mental retardation – hence the acronym WAGR. Cytogenetic analysis of patients with WAGR syndrome showed deletions of chromosome 11 centered around 11p13. Loss of heterozygosity for 11p markers has been demonstrated in Wilms tumors. Confirmation of the suppressive nature of a gene in this area was shown by the observation that a Wilms tumor cell line could no longer produce tumors in nude mice following the introduction of a normal chromosome 11 by microcell fusion.

Comparison of constitutional deletions in patients with Wilms tumor, using cloned probes, narrowed the critical region containing the gene to between the catalase gene and the gene for the follicle-stimulating hormone beta sub-unit at 11p13. The region has been resolved further into an aniridia locus at a more telomeric position, and a locus involved in genito-urinary abnormalities and Wilms tumor at a more centromeric position. A candidate for a Wilms tumor gene has recently been isolated by means of reverse genetics. The gene encodes a zinc finger protein probably involved in the control of transcription [13]. This candidate gene is expressed in tissues of the developing kidney, the genital ridge, fetal gonad and mesothelium and is therefore involved in genito-urinary development [14].

It is possible that two other genes in this region play a role in the development of the tumor. Beckwith–Wiedemann Syndrome (BWS) is characterized by exomphalos, macroglossia and gigantism; it also carries an increased risk of developing tumors, especially Wilms tumor. Most cases are sporadic but families have been described in which the disease segregates as an autosomal dominant trait. Abnormalities of 11p have been found in a number of patients, but particularly affecting band 11p15 rather than 11p13. Tight linkage to 11p15 markers has been demonstrated in a family with BWS. Loss of heterozygosity of markers distal to the 11p13 region has been found in tumors associated with BWS such as rhabdomyosarcoma. Consequently, a second locus involved in BWS and distinct from that at 11p13 has been implicated at 11p15 [15]. Genetic linkage to 11p13 and 11p15 has been excluded in two Wilms tumor families, implying a third locus outside this region [16].

### 2.2.2 Familial adenomatous polyposis

Familial adenomatous polyposis (FAP) is characterized clinically by the presence of hundreds to thousands of polyps throughout the colon and rectum (*Figure 2.8*) and at least one of these will become malignant from the second decade of life onwards. The observation of a cytogenetically detectable deletion in a patient with FAP led to the localization of the gene, termed the *APC* gene (for adenomatous polyposis coli), to chromosome 5q21 by family linkage studies (see Chapter 5). The *APC* gene is believed to be a tumor suppressor gene but it may act differently from that described in retinoblastoma. Carcinomas arising in FAP patients frequently show loss of heterozygosity of chromosome 5q markers (20–30%) but allele loss in the adenomas is rare. The inheritance of a single mutant *APC* gene is therefore

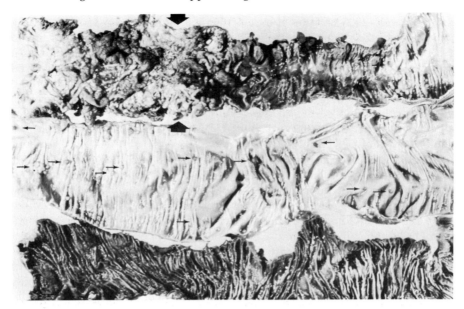

**Figure 2.8:** *A resected colon and rectum from a 21-year-old female with FAP showing a Dukes C adenocarcinoma (large arrows) and multiple polyps (small arrows) throughout. Figure courtesy of Dr J. Newman, Histopathology Department, East Birmingham Hospital, U.K.*

sufficient for the development of polyps, possibly by giving the epithelial cells a proliferative advantage. The *APC* gene may normally act as a negative regulator of colonic epithelial proliferation. The loss of one allele is sufficient to decrease levels of the gene product such that efficient control of cell proliferation is no longer possible [17]. Thus, the idea of tumor suppressor genes acting in a recessive manner through loss of alleles on both chromosomes is not always as clear cut as early studies suggested.

In FAP, as in sporadic cancers (see below), other genes – both oncogenes and tumor suppressor genes – have been shown to act, confirming once again that carcinogenesis, whether hereditary or sporadic, is a multistage process. In cases of FAP, these various events take place over 30–40 years. In sporadic cancers, six to seven decades are required before these events accumulate. The mutation in the *APC* gene may therefore give the tumor a 'head start'.

### 2.2.3 Neurofibromatosis 1

Von Recklinghausen neurofibromatosis (NF1) is an autosomal dominant disorder characterized by *café au lait* spots, multiple neurofibromas and an increased risk of cancer. It has been associated – probably erroneously – with the Elephant Man, Joseph Merrick. The disease has been localized to chromosome 17 by linkage analysis and also by the cytogenetic observation of translocations involving 17q11. Several candidate genes for NF1 were proposed including two oncogenes, *ERBA1* and *ERBB2* (*NEU*) and nerve growth factor receptor. However, these were all excluded either because individuals were identified who had a recombination between the candidate gene and *NF1* or through physical mapping studies [18]. Rapid progress in this field has meant that the *NF1* gene has recently been cloned [19]. Northern blots indicate that the mRNA is at least 13 kb. The very high mutation rate for this disease – about 50% of cases are new mutations – suggested that the gene would turn out to be large. Evidence now indicates that it is likely to cover at least 250 kb of the genome. Interestingly, several other small genes transcribed in the opposite orientation have been found in the introns of the *NF1* gene. It is not yet clear whether these play any part in the disease. Preliminary evidence suggests that *NF1* shares sequence homology with the mammalian GAP protein.

Neurofibromas themselves are polyclonal in origin, making it impossible to look for loss of heterozygosity. A high frequency of chromosome 17 loss has been described in neurofibrosarcomas but as there is already a suppressor gene on 17p (*p53*; see Section 2.3), the analysis has proven complicated because the loss has generally involved the whole chromosome. It therefore remains to be seen whether the *NF1* gene is a tumor suppressor.

### 2.2.4 Other hereditary cancers associated with tumor suppressor genes

Other diseases associated with cancers and which show a hereditary form are listed in *Table 2.1*. In some cases, such as bilateral acoustic neurofibromatosis (NF2), allele loss was found on chromosome 22 in meningiomas and neurofibromas from patients with NF2. This prompted linkage analysis with chromosome 22 probes and led to the mapping of the disease to 22q. In other cases such as MEN2A which is mapped to chromosome 10, loss of heterozygosity was seen in chromosomes 1 and 22. This suggests that genes on chromosomes 1 and 22 may co-operate with the MEN2A gene on chromosome 10 in tumorigenesis.

**Table 2.1:** *Loss of heterozygosity in inherited cancers*

| Disease | Tumor | Site of gene | LOH[a] |
|---------|-------|--------------|--------|
| FAP | Colorectal | 5q21–22 | 5q21–22<br>17p |
| MEN1 | Anterior pituitary<br>insulinomas | 11q12–13 | 11 |
| MEN2A | Medullary thyroid<br>carcinoma<br>Phaeochromocytoma<br>Parathyroid adenoma | 10p12-q11 | 1p<br>and<br>22q |
| NF1 | Neurofibrosarcomas | 17q11 | 17q |
| NF2 | Schwannomas | 22q | 22q |
| Retinoblastoma | Retinoblastoma | 13q14 | 13q14 |
| Von Hippel Lindau | Renal cell cancer | 3p | |
| Wilms tumor | Wilms tumor | 11p13 | 11p13 |

[a] LOH = loss of heterozygosity.

## 2.3 *p53*

The *p53* gene is located on the short arm of chromosome 17. It is made up of 11 exons covering 16–20 kb of DNA and encodes a 2.2–2.5 kb mRNA producing a 53 kd nuclear protein. This protein is found in most cells of the body and has a short half-life. Much is already known about the gene since its identification over 10 years ago. The reasons are twofold: (a) it has properties of both a tumor suppressor gene and an oncogene and therefore is intrinsically interesting, (b) it is found mutated and/or deleted in a wide range and number of tumors and is therefore likely to play an important role in tumorigenesis [20].

### 2.3.1 p53 *as an oncogene*

Many mutations (point mutations, insertions and deletions) have been shown to occur over an extensive region of the gene, all of which cause its activation.

Mutant forms of *p53* can immortalize primary rat fibroblasts in culture. Together with the *RAS* oncogene, *p53* will produce transformed foci in rat embryo fibroblasts in culture whereas neither is capable of doing so alone. Transfected *p53* can also increase the tumorigenicity of established cell lines and convert untransformed lines to a more malignant phenotype. In transformed cells, the protein has an extended half-life resulting in elevated levels in the cells. In cell lines transformed by SV40 virus or adenovirus, the p53 protein is found complexed to the SV40 tumor antigen or the adenovirus E1b protein, respectively. It is these complexes which increase the half-life of the protein resulting in elevated levels in virally transformed cells. It is also found associated with heat-shock proteins and by virtue of this association is found in the cytoplasm as well as the nucleus. This high level of *p53* gene product is essential for efficient transformation.

### 2.3.2 p53 *as a tumor suppressor gene*

A consistent deletion of the short arm of chromosome 17 has been seen in many tumors (*Table 2.2*). A study of brain, breast, lung and colon tumors showed that in the majority of cases where *p53* was deleted there was a detectable mutation in the remaining *p53* allele [21]. This picture of a deletion plus mutation of the remaining allele is the hallmark of tumor suppressor genes as described earlier for the hereditary tumors. The oncogene/suppressor gene

**Table 2.2:** *Tumors with deletions of 17p*

| | |
|---|---|
| Adrenal cortical tumors | Lung tumors |
| Bladder cancer | Neurofibrosarcomas |
| Brain tumors | Osteosarcomas |
| Breast cancer | Ovarian cancer |
| Cervical cancer | Renal cell cancer |
| Colorectal tumors | Testicular tumors |
| Hepatocellular cancer | |

effect is explained by the observation that the mutant *p53* complexes with wild-type protein and possibly heat-shock proteins to create an inactive complex. Therefore mutant *p53* causes tumor progression by a dominant negative effect. Further loss of growth control might be expected if the wild-type allele is subsequently deleted, leaving the cell with one mutant allele. An example of this intermediate step has been shown in one example of a colorectal tumor. This tumor had a mutation in *p53* but still produced the wild-type protein as well as the mutant form. It was suggested that if the tumor had not been removed, loss of the wild-type would be the next step leading to tumor progression [21]. This loss of 17p alleles has indeed been shown to be associated with tumor progression in man. In some families where breast cancer segregates as a Mendelian dominant condition (Li–Fraumeni Syndrome), a mutation in the *p53* gene is transmitted through the germ-line. This is similar to the transmission of a mutant *RB1* gene in familial retinoblastoma.

## 2.4 Evidence for tumor suppressor genes in sporadic cancers

Comparison of the results of allele loss in hereditary cancers with that seen in sporadic cancers, for example, between FAP and colorectal cancer, has suggested that the fundamental mechanism for carcinogenesis may be the same for both. Many sporadic cancers have been examined for loss of hetero-zygosity and *Table 2.3* gives an overview of those tumors in which allele loss has been demonstrated. It is still not clear whether all these regions contain tumor suppressor genes.

It is apparent that in many tumors more than one chromosomal region is involved. This is only to be expected if we imagine tumors to arise via a multi-stage process involving several genes. *Table 2.3* also shows that there is no particular tissue specificity for the tumor suppressor genes. Loss of 17p, presumably involving *p53*, has, for example, been implicated in a wide range of tumors and the prototype tumor suppressor *RB1* has been mutated in such diverse tumors as small cell lung cancer (SCLC), breast cancer and hemato-logical malignancies.

**Table 2.3:** *Allele loss in human tumors*

| Tumor | Chromosomal region lost |
|---|---|
| Bladder | 2p, 3p, 11p |
| Breast | 1q, 3p, 11p, 13q, 17p, 17q |
| Colon | All chromosomes except 2 |
| Lung | 3p, 11p, 13q, 17p |
| Ovary | 11p |
| Stomach | 13, 18q |
| Testicular | 11p, 17p |

## 2.5 Interaction and differences between oncogenes and tumor suppressor genes

As mentioned in Chapter 1 and alluded to at various points in this chapter, no single genetic event causes tumors. Even retinoblastoma, which has been described as being caused by mutations in a single gene, does not contradict this because at least two hits are required in the gene for the tumor to develop. Other oncogenes, for example, *MYCN*, have also been shown to contribute to the development of retinoblastomas. Colorectal cancer has been studied perhaps more than any other tumor when investigating the ways in which tumor suppressor genes and oncogenes might interact, and as such serves as a good model for other cancers.

**Table 2.4:** *Inherited syndromes associated with colorectal cancer*

---

Cancer family
Familial adenomatous polyposis
Gorlin's basal cell nevus
Juvenile polyposis
Muir Torre
Peutz-Jegher
Site-specific colon cancer
Turcot's

---

### 2.5.1 Interaction between oncogenes and suppressor genes – the colorectal cancer model

Colorectal cancer has several hereditary forms (*Table 2.4*) which have given some clues as to the genes involved in the development of sporadic forms of the cancer. It also has a well-defined pattern of progression (*Figure 2.9*). For these reasons, and also because it is one of the commonest forms of cancer, more is known about colorectal cancer than most other sporadic cancers. *Table 2.5* shows the major changes in oncogenes and tumor suppressor genes seen in colorectal cancer [22]. *RAS* has been discussed in Chapter 1 and the *APC* gene and *p53* in this chapter. The *DCC* gene (deleted in colorectal cancer) has recently been identified following the observation of a high rate of allele loss on chromosome 18q which suggested the existence of a tumor suppressor. The *DCC* gene encodes a protein which is similar in sequence to neural cell adhesion molecules and other related cell surface glycoproteins. It is present in most normal tissues but its expression is reduced or absent in the

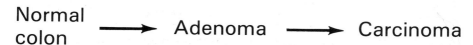

**Figure 2.9:** *Pattern of development of colorectal cancer.*

***Table 2.5:*** *Involvement of oncogenes and tumor suppressor genes in sporadic colorectal cancer*

| Gene | Location | Percentage of adenomas | | | Percentage of cancers |
| | | Early | Intermediate | Late | |
|------|----------|-------|--------------|------|----------------------|
| *APC* | 5q21 | 0 | 30 | 30 | 20–50 |
| *DCC* | 18q | 13 | 11 | 47 | 70 |
| *KRAS* | 12q | 10 | 50 | 50 | 50 |
| *p53* | 17p | 6 | 6 | 24 | 75 |

Data from [22] and personal communications.

majority of colorectal cancers. Its role in the development of colorectal cancers is probably via alterations in the regulation of cell to cell contact [22].

These alterations have been put together to suggest a model for tumorigenesis as shown in *Figure 2.10* [22]. Other oncogenes, for example, *MYC*, tumor suppressor genes, for example, *RB1*, and loss of other chromosome regions – 1q, 4p, 6p, 6q, 8p, 9q and 22q – have also been seen in colorectal cancers and may be involved at various stages. In addition, other epigenetic phenomena such as loss of methyl groups have been shown to occur early in tumorigenesis and may contribute to the instability of the genome. This colorectal model is similar to that described for other tumors such as SCLC, breast cancer and melanoma where, again, preliminary evidence for interactions between oncogenes and tumor suppressor genes has been observed. Such a model provides us with a framework on which to expand.

### 2.5.2 Differences between oncogenes and tumor suppressor genes

Initially it was believed that these two types of genes behaved in different ways. Oncogenes were believed to act in a dominant manner, only one copy being required for tumor formation. Tumor suppressor genes were believed to

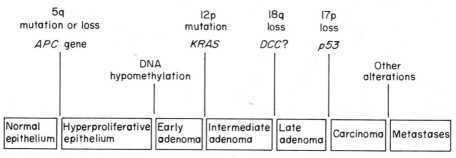

***Figure 2.10:*** *Model for the interaction of oncogenes and tumor suppressor genes in colorectal tumorigenesis. Figure reproduced from [22] with permission from Cell Press.*

be recessive in nature, with deletion of both copies necessary for tumorigenesis. This division is now seen as false. For example, loss of only one copy of the *APC* gene is necessary for formation of polyps in FAP. *p53* is known to behave both as an oncogene and as a tumor suppressor. Even the classic oncogene, *RAS*, and tumor suppressor gene, *RB1*, do not behave 'correctly'. The tumorigenic phenotype of rat fibroblasts transformed by *HRAS* is suppressed by subsequent transfection of the normal *HRAS* gene. Alterations of *RB1* without deletion of the normal allele have been identified in a number of tumors such as breast and lung. Our theories of how oncogenes and tumor suppressor genes operate therefore have to remain flexible [23].

## 2.6 Function of tumor suppressor genes

The functions of many tumor suppressor genes have not yet been identified, but several areas in which the genes may be involved are shown in *Table 2.6* [23]. Several tumor suppressor genes have had specific roles identified. Both *RB1* and *p53* are known to bind DNA and have been shown to act at specific stages of the cell cycle. One possible function may therefore be to act as negative regulators of growth by controlling transcription of cell-cycle dependent genes. Similarly, the Wilms tumor gene has been hypothesized to act by switching genes off or on during the normal development of the kidney. Once mutated in tumors, it can no longer regulate its target genes, leading to uncontrolled proliferation with aberrant differentiation and eventual tumor formation [14].

Involvement of the *DCC* gene in cell to cell contact has already been described. This physical contact between cells is important for the control of cell growth. Other genes involved in this function may therefore also prove to act as tumor suppressors.

Transforming growth factor β (TGF-β) inhibits the proliferation of a wide range of cells, particularly epithelial cells, by binding to a cell surface receptor. Similar properties are shared with tumor necrosis factor and the interferons [23].

Finally, in somatic cell hybrids, malignancy appears to be suppressed either by the imposition of the terminal differentiation pattern of the normal partner on the malignant cell, or by complementation of a defect which impairs differentiation in the malignant cell. Tumor suppressors may therefore play a role in cell differentiation [24].

These are just a few examples where the function of a tumor suppressor gene is known. At the present time the mechanism by which others work remains the topic of intensive research.

***Table 2.6***: *Possible functions of tumor suppressor genes*

Affect differentiation
Control of cell to cell contact, e.g. *DCC*
Growth inhibitory factors, e.g. TGF-β
Interact with oncogenes, e.g. *p53*
Regulation of transcription, e.g. *RB1, p53* and Wilms gene

# References

1. Harris, H. (1988) *Cancer Res.*, **48**, 3302.
2. Stanbridge, E.J. (1986) *BioEssays*, **3**, 252.
3. Knudson, A.G. Jr. (1971) *Proc. Natl Acad. Sci. U.S.A.*, **68**, 820.
4. Benedict, W.F., Banerjee, A., Mark, C. and Murphree, A.L. (1982) *Cancer Genet. Cytogenet.*, **6**, 213.
5. Knudson, A.G. Jr. (1985) *Cancer Res.*, **45**, 1437.
6. Cavenee, W.K., Dryja, T.P., Phillips, R.A., Benedict, W.F., Godbout, R., Gallie, B.L., Murphree, A.L., Strong, L.C. and White, R.L. (1983) *Nature*, **305**, 779.
7. Friend, S.H., Bernards, R., Rogelj, S., Weinberg, R.A., Rapaport, J.M., Albert, D.M. and Dryja, T.P. (1986) *Nature*, **323**, 643.
8. Lee, W.H., Bookstein, R., Hong, F., Yoing, L.J., Shew, J.H. and Lee, E.Y.H.P. (1987) *Science*, **235**, 1394.
9. Fung, Y.K.T., Murphree, A.L., T'ang, A., Qian, J., Hinrichs, H.S. and Benedict, W.F. (1987) *Science*, **236**, 1657.
10. Lee, W.W., Shew, J.Y., Hong, F.D., Sery, T.W., Donoso, L.A., Young, L.J., Bookstein, R. and Lee, E.Y.H.P. (1987) *Nature*, **329**, 642.
11. Channing, S. and Dryja, T. (1989) *Proc. Natl Acad. Sci. U.S.A.*, **86**, 5044.
12. Matsunaga, E. (1981) *Hum. Genet.*, **57**, 231.
13. Gessler, M., Poustka, A., Cavenee, W., Neve, R.L., Orkin, S.H. and Bruns, G.A.P. (1990) *Nature*, **343**, 774.
14. Pritchard-Jones, K., Fleming, S., Davidson, D. *et al.* (1990) *Nature*, **346**, 194.
15. Koufos, A., Grundy, P., Morgan, K., Aleck, K.A., Hadro, T., Lampkin, B.C., Kalbakji, A. and Cavanee, W.K. (1989) *Am. J. Hum. Genet.*, **44**, 711.
16. Grundy, P., Koufos, A., Morgan, K., Li, F.P., Meadows, A.T. and Cavenee, W.K. (1988) *Nature*, **336**, 374.
17. Bodmer, W.F., Bailey, C.J., Bodmer, J. *et al.* (1987) *Nature*, **328**, 614.
18. Collins, F.S., Ponder, B.A.J., Seizinger, B.R. and Epstein, C.J. (1989) *Am. J. Hum. Genet.*, **44**, 1.
19. Wallace, M.R., Marchuk, D.A., Andersen, L.B. *et al.* (1990) *Science*, **249**, 181.
20. Levine, A.J. (1990) *BioEssays*, **12**, 60.
21. Nigro, J.M., Baker, S.J., Preisinger, A.C. *et al.* (1989) *Nature*, **342**, 705.
22. Fearon, E.R. and Vogelstein, B. (1990) *Cell*, **61**, 759.
23. Steel, C.M. (1989) *Proc. R. Coll. Phys. Edin.*, **19**, 413.
24. Paul, J. (1989) *Histopathology*, **15**, 1.

# Note added in proof

A candidate gene for a tumor suppressor gene located at 5q21 – possibly the *APC* gene – has recently been identified [Kinzler, K.W. *et al.* (1991), *Science*, **251**, 1366]. So far mutations in this gene have been found in three cases of sporadic colorectal cancer. Two of the mutations are point mutations and the third is a deletion. No mutations have as yet been identified in tumors from FAP patients.

# 3
# TECHNIQUES FOR THE ANALYSIS OF ONCOGENES AND TUMOR SUPPRESSOR GENES

An understanding of the methodology used in the analysis of oncogenes and tumor suppressor genes is fundamental to understanding how these genes can be used for the diagnosis and prognosis of cancer. There are many excellent molecular biology textbooks available which describe these procedures in detail [1,2]. This chapter outlines these techniques briefly so that those unfamiliar with the technology can follow the subsequent chapters without immediate recourse to other books.

Oncogenes and tumor suppressor genes can be studied at three levels, namely DNA, RNA or protein. These molecules can be either within the cell in prepared tissue sections (*in situ*) or in isolation. These two approaches give different information. Isolated DNA can be examined for qualitative and quantitative abnormalities. This is useful when looking for rearrangements or mutations within a particular gene and also for assessing absolute levels of a gene (gene amplification). Analysis of isolated RNA gives information about the level of transcription (gene expression). Direct analysis of protein allows the determination of protein levels or of changes in protein size.

*In-situ* analysis provides information concerning the spatial distribution of these molecules in the cell and therefore shows which cells are expressing a particular gene, RNA sequence or protein molecule, but cannot easily be used for quantitative analysis.

## 3.1 Analysis of DNA or RNA

### 3.1.1 Southern blotting

Once any segment of DNA has been cloned and characterized, copies can then be used as probes to identify variation in the DNA composition of a study population. One widely used technique is termed Southern blotting – not for any geographical reason but because it was developed by Professor

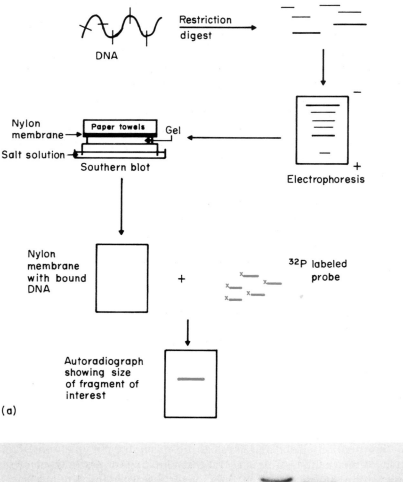

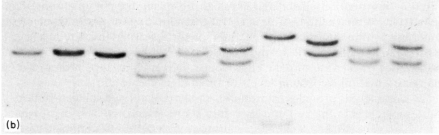

**Figure 3.1:** *(a) Southern blotting technique. (b) Example of the end-product of Southern blotting – an autoradiograph showing bands of different sizes corresponding to the different RFLPs.*

E. Southern in the 1970s. All techniques subsequently developed for the analysis of RNA or protein have, however, continued this analogy, hence, Northern (RNA), Western (protein) and even South-western (DNA/protein) blotting.

The basis of Southern blotting is shown in *Figure 3.1*. DNA is extracted from the tissues or cells and digested into small fragments with restriction enzymes. These enzymes, which are isolated from bacteria, selectively cut DNA at sites dependent on specific nucleotide sequences in the genome (restriction sites; *Table 3.1*). Following digestion, these double-stranded DNA fragments are separated according to size by electrophoresis on an agarose gel. Treatment of the DNA in the gel with alkali produces single-stranded molecules, which are transferred or 'blotted' onto nitrocellulose or nylon membranes. The presence or absence of sequences of interest is then determined by incubating the membrane with the relevant DNA probe which has previously been radiolabeled (usually with $^{32}$P) and made single-stranded. Hybridization between the complementary sequences of the probe and target DNA is detected by autoradiography, allowing recognition of the DNA sequence under investigation and assessment of alterations in its size, copy number, etc. [1].

**Table 3.1:** *Commonly used restriction enzymes*

| Name | Recognition sequence | Bacterial strain of origin |
|------|----------------------|----------------------------|
| *Bam*HI | GGATCC<br>CCTAGG | *Bacillus amyloliquefaciens* |
| *Eco*RI | GAATTC<br>CTTAAG | *Escherichia coli* |
| *Hind*III | AAGCTT<br>TTCGAA | *Hemophilus influenzae* |
| *Pst*I | CTGCAG<br>GACGTC | *Providencia stuartii* |
| *Taq*I | TCGA<br>AGCT | *Thermus aquaticus* |

### 3.1.2 Northern blotting

This technique is essentially the same as Southern blotting except that intact messenger RNA (mRNA) is separated on the gels and again detected, following blotting, by probing with a radiolabeled DNA fragment. This allows the amount of the transcript to be determined and can also be used to detect abnormalities in the size of the mRNA [1].

### 3.1.3 Polymerase chain reaction

In 1985, a technique allowing specific amplification of selected sequences of DNA was described. This polymerase chain reaction (PCR) technique relies on a knowledge of at least part of the DNA sequence around the region of interest, because short specific oligonucleotides complementary to sequences either side of this region are required to prime the synthesis of the DNA sequence between them. The process involves three stages: denaturation of the double-stranded DNA, annealing of the oligonucleotide primers, and synthesis of DNA by a thermostable DNA polymerase. By repeating the process 20–30 times, up to several million copies of the DNA can be made (*Figure 3.2*). The main advantages of this technique are (a) it is rapid, particularly as the product can often be detected directly on agarose gels; this takes

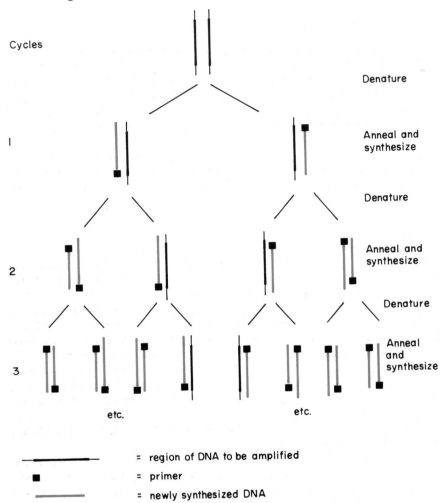

**Figure 3.2:** *Polymerase chain reaction.*

several hours to perform, unlike Southern blotting which can take several days or more, and (b) it is extremely sensitive; it is possible to start with a single molecule of DNA and finish with sufficient for analysis [3].

A further refinement of this technique involves the hybridization of the PCR product with oligonucleotide probes specific for a known mutation, such as the point mutation in the *RAS* oncogene. This technique has been used successfully to analyze the distribution of *RAS* mutations in different tissues [4].

PCR is also a very useful technique for the production of single-stranded DNA which can be sequenced directly and it has been used in this way to investigate point mutations in the *p53* gene on chromosome 17.

### 3.1.4 In-situ *hybridization*

This technique permits the direct analysis of sequences of DNA or RNA in tissues so that specific cells, populations of cells, or chromosomes can be examined [5]. The method involves the denaturation of DNA in a tissue section followed by the application of a labeled probe which is complementary to the sequence of interest. As with Southern blotting it is possible to use a radioactively labeled probe but here the isotopes used are usually $^3$H, $^{125}$I or $^{35}$S (*Figure 3.3*).

In addition, it is now common to use probes labeled with biotin which can be detected by an enzymatic reaction. This technique has several advantages over radioisotopes, particularly safety and the long-term stability of the labeled probe.

### 3.1.5 RFLP analysis

Approximately every 200 bp along the length of the chromosomes the sequence of DNA varies between individuals. These sites usually alter by only a single base change. Where they coincide with restriction sites the alteration can be detected by restriction enzymes. The presence or absence of any particular site is variable in the population, hence the term polymorphism. The variation does not usually confer any phenotypic effect since the variations are frequently found in introns rather than coding exons. In the example shown in *Figure 3.4*, if the DNA from individuals with different DNA polymorphisms is digested with a restriction enzyme and then Southern blotted, individuals with chromosome A will have a 5 kb fragment detected by the probe, whereas individuals with chromosome B will have a 3 kb fragment detected by the same probe. The 5 kb fragment is arbitrarily called allele 1 and the 3 kb fragment allele 2.

These RFLPs can be very useful markers and have been used successfully for the diagnosis of many single gene disorders such as Duchenne muscular dystrophy or cystic fibrosis. In cancer research they have been used in two different areas: (a) RFLPs have been detected in and around oncogenes and particular alleles have been shown to have prognostic significance, and (b) they have been used to track the defective gene in families with inherited cancers such as FAP.

For the detection of inherited diseases, the basis of the test is as follows: DNA from individuals in a family is digested with restriction enzymes and subjected to Southern blotting as described earlier. Each individual in the family is then given a genotype corresponding to the alleles present on either of the two chromosomes. *Figure 3.5* shows the result for three individuals using the probe and RFLP shown in *Figure 3.4*. Individual 1 is homozygous for allele 1, that is, has two copies of chromosome A. Individual 3 is also homozygous, but this time for allele 2. The individual shown in the center is a heterozygote, that is, has one copy of chromosome A and one of chromosome B. By entering these results on to the family pedigree along with results from any other members of the family available, it is possible to determine which allele, corresponding to a particular restriction fragment length, segregates

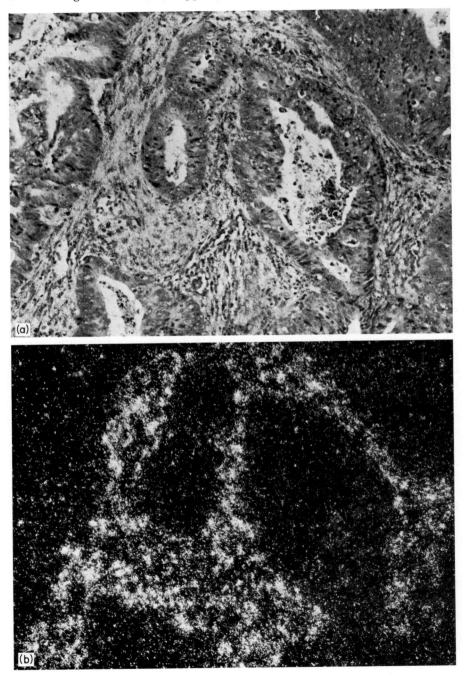

**Figure 3.3:** *(a) Paraffin section of a colon cancer. Bright-field illumination to show tissue morphology. (b) In-situ hybridization using a $^{35}$S-labeled cDNA probe to detect type 1 collagen mRNA. Detection is by autoradiography. Dark-field illumination to show silver grain distribution. Photographs courtesy of D.G. Powe, G.I. Carter and R.E. Hewitt, Department of Histopathology, University of Nottingham, Nottingham, U.K.*

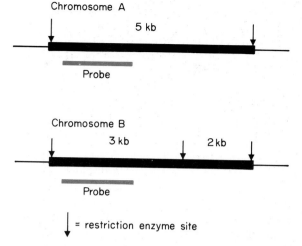

**Figure 3.4:** *Example of a RFLP showing one chromosome with a 5 kb DNA fragment and a second chromosome with a 3 kb fragment recognized by the same probe. Arrows indicate the restriction sites.*

with the disease allele for that particular pedigree. In the pedigree shown in *Figure 3.6*, of an autosomal dominant disease such as FAP, the results suggest that allele 2 is segregating with the disease in this particular family. This is suggested because the affected individual (II-3) has inherited the chromosome with allele 2 from her affected mother, whereas her normal brother and sister have inherited the normal chromosome carrying allele 1 from their mother. By examination of this pedigree one important point can be seen: the presence or absence of a particular allele does not in itself signify that an individual is affected or normal. In *Figure 3.6*, individual I-3, who has married into this family, has two copies of allele 2 and is normal. The RFLP is merely a marker which can be used to follow the pattern of inheritance of a particular chromosome through a family. The second important point to make about this type of analysis is that because many of the RFLPs are located around the disease gene rather than in it, there is the possiblity during meiosis of a crossover in the DNA between the RFLP and the gene. The further away the RFLP, the higher the chance of such a recombination until ultimately it is so

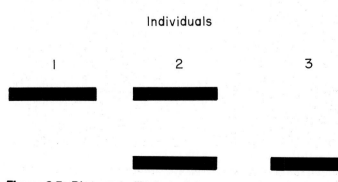

**Figure 3.5:** *Diagram to illustrate the patterns of bands seen in three individuals following Southern blotting and hybridization with the probe described in* Figure *3.4. Individuals 1 and 3 are homozygous for the 5 kb and 3 kb fragments, respectively, and individual 2 is a heterozygote.*

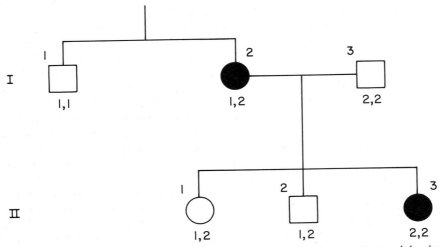

**Figure 3.6**: *Pedigree of a family with a disease segregating in an autosomal dominant manner (see text for detailed explanation of results). The genotypes associated with the RFLPs described in Figures 3.4 and 3.5 are shown.*

far away that it cannot be used for the analysis. All results of such a test have to carry with them an error rate to take account of the possibility of such a recombination event.

## 3.2 Analysis of proteins

An alternative strategy used to examine the expression of oncogenes is to look at the oncoproteins themselves rather than at the DNA or RNA. This method has some advantages. In particular, it means that a retrospective analysis of tumor material can be made. This is made possible by the availability of paraffin blocks from surgically resected specimens. This material is not suitable for analysis of RNA – although it is now possible to extract DNA from the blocks for analysis by PCR. The presence of oncoproteins in such tissue is most easily assessed by the application of antibodies. The most obvious advantage of this technique is the ability to test samples from individuals for whom the clinical outcome is known. In studies of the value of oncogenes as prognostic indicators this is invaluable as prospective studies could take years to perform. In order to study oncoprotein expression, however, antibodies have to be produced.

### 3.2.1 Production of antibodies to oncoproteins

In general, antibodies to the oncoproteins have been raised against synthetic peptides rather than the native protein molecule. Short peptides, synthesized on the basis of known DNA sequences and coupled to protein carriers, have been used as immunogens. The region chosen for synthesis of the peptides is selected following the construction of a hydrophobicity plot and includes those residues thought to be exposed on the surface of the intact molecule. Both monoclonal and polyclonal antibodies have been produced in this way and the approach has found many useful applications [6].

A number of antibodies have been produced to the *RAS* p21 protein. Some of these antibodies are reactive with both normal and mutant forms of the protein, for example, Y13 259, whereas others have been raised to a peptide containing the amino acid sequence corresponding to one of the forms of activated *RAS* and are specific for the mutated form of p21 [7]. A third antibody (RAP 5) has also been raised to a peptide reflecting the amino acid sequence of one of the activated forms of *RAS* but it cross-reacts with both the normal and mutated form of p21 [8]. Some care has to be taken when interpreting the results of studies using these antibodies, because the antigenic target for some of them remains controversial. Several antibodies (Myc1-6E10 and Myc1-9E10) to the *MYC* oncoprotein have been produced in a similar way, and again on further characterization it appears that one of these, Myc1-6E10, may not recognize the product of the *MYC* gene [9].

A final novel approach to producing antibodies specific for tumor cells has been to transfect the NIH-3T3 cell line with DNA fragments obtained from a human acute lymphocytic leukemia (ALL) and to use the transformants as immunogens to raise antibodies. Although the antigen has not been characterized in detail, at least one antibody produced in this way did not react with NIH-3T3 or with the majority of normal tissues tested but did react with certain tumors, including ALLs and sarcomas [10].

A list of some of the antibodies to oncoproteins currently available is shown in *Table 3.2*. The potential for the use of these antibodies is great, not only for examining the expression of the proteins in tissues but also for monitoring the levels of oncoproteins in body fluids and as potential carriers of therapeutic agents to cells – the so-called 'magic bullets'. Some of their applications are discussed in Chapter 4 and the techniques used in their study are described in the following sections, but on the whole the potential of the antibodies to the oncoproteins has not yet been fully realized.

**Table 3.2:** *Oncogenes for which antibodies to oncoproteins are currently available*

| | |
|---|---|
| ABL | ERBB1 |
| ERBB2 | FMS |
| FOS | HRAS |
| KRAS | MOS |
| MYB | MYC |
| NRAS | SIS |

Note: this list is not comprehensive.

### 3.2.2 Western blotting

An overall examination of the size and quantity of oncoproteins in cells is possible by the technique of Western blotting. Proteins are extracted from cells and separated on polyacrylamide gels on the basis of size and/or charge. They are then transferred to nitrocellulose or nylon membranes. Unlike

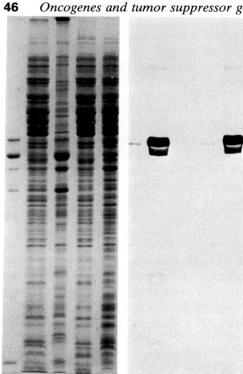

**Figure 3.7:** *(a) Polyacrylamide gel stained for total proteins and (b) Western blot of proteins extracted from tumor cells reacted with a monoclonal antibody to a tumor marker.*

Southern blotting, transfer of proteins by passive diffusion is inefficient; Western blotting requires the application of an electric current for several hours. Following transfer, the protein of interest can be detected by incubation of the membrane in an antibody solution followed by detection with an enzymatically labeled second antibody [11] (*Figure 3.7*).

### 3.2.3 Immunocytochemical techniques

Immunocytochemical techniques are used widely throughout all areas of research to study expression of proteins in tissues, essentially by applying antibodies to thin sections of tissues – either frozen sections or sections of tissue which have been fixed and embedded in paraffin wax. Antibodies may be labeled directly with an enzyme such as horseradish peroxidase or alkaline phosphatase. Their binding sites can then be visualized by incubation of the tissue with a substrate which yields a colored product. More commonly, a second enzymatically labeled antibody specific for the primary antibody is used; this technique is described schematically in *Figure 3.8*. A typical result showing the distribution of the *MYC* oncoprotein in a section of gastric carcinoma is illustrated in *Figure 3.9*.

### 3.2.4 Flow cytometry

The development of the fluorescence-activated cell sorter (FACS) has provided an alternative method of studying oncogene expression – a method

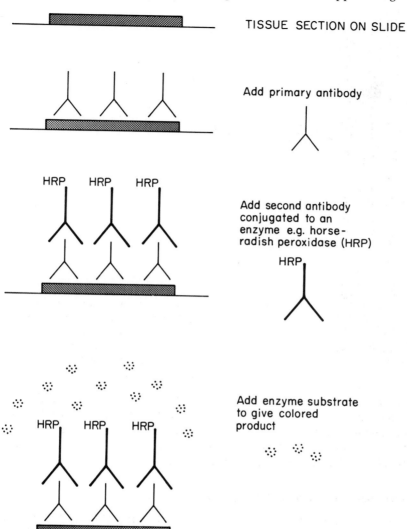

TISSUE SECTION ON SLIDE

Add primary antibody

Add second antibody
conjugated to an
enzyme e.g. horse-
radish peroxidase (HRP)

HRP

Add enzyme substrate
to give colored
product

**Figure 3.8:** *Flow diagram to illustrate the immunohistochemical technique.*

often referred to as flow cytometry. A wide range of particles can be analyzed
using the FACS, including whole cells, nuclei, chromosomes, bacteria, etc.
Regardless of what is to be analyzed, the process is essentially the same. The
particles are labeled with an appropriate fluorochrome and then passed individually through a laser beam. The emitted light for each individual particle
is collected, measured and stored on computer. Other information such as
particle volume and a measure of the granularity of particles can also be
collected. In addition to the analysis, individual particles expressing particular
pre-set parameters, such as fluorescence intensity, can be deflected electro-
statically into collection tubes so that they can be analyzed further at the end
of the experiment [12] (*Figure 3.10*). The fluorochrome used can be a fluores-
cent dye, such as fluorescein, coupled to an antibody specific for the protein

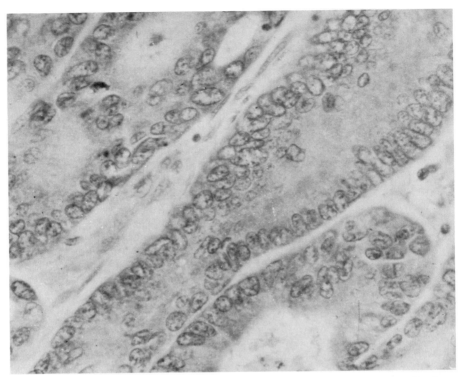

***Figure 3.9:*** *Example of a section of a gastric carcinoma reacted with an antibody to p62, showing cytoplasmic staining.*

under investigation, or it can be a nucleic-acid specific stain such as propidium iodide, ethidium bromide or DAPI. The whole procedure is extremely rapid with thousands of particles being analyzed every second. A wide variety of parameters can subsequently be plotted either individually or against each other from the information obtained (*Figure 3.11*).

Nuclear oncogenes such as *MYC* and *FOS* have been extensively studied using flow cytometry [13]. Nuclei for analysis can be extracted from fresh tissues but can also be obtained from paraffin blocks. By dual labeling with a fluorochrome-labeled antibody plus a DNA-specific stain, it is possible to correlate the DNA content (ploidy status) with the expression of an oncogene in individual cells. The detection of aneuploidy in some tumors has been shown to correlate with a worse prognosis. The technique of combining information on oncogene expression with ploidy status may enhance its prognostic significance.

Flow cytometry is a very rapid method of determining the expression of oncoproteins on a cell by cell or nucleus by nucleus basis. It also has the advantage that, like immunohistochemical staining techniques, archival material can be used to obtain prognostic information. One drawback in the study of nuclei obtained from archival material, in addition to the problems previously mentioned concerning the specificity of the antibodies, is the apparent loss of reactivity of the nuclear antigens because of the harsh

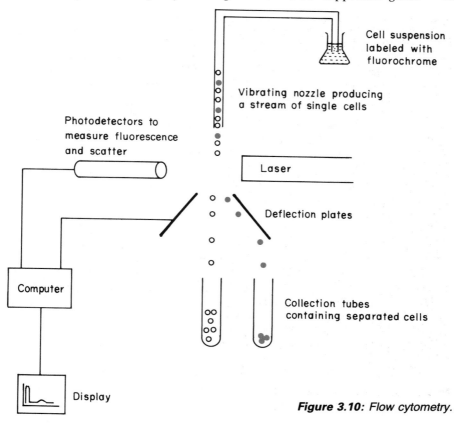

**Figure 3.10:** Flow cytometry.

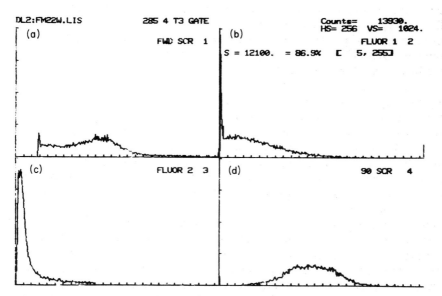

**Figure 3.11:** Parameters measured by flow cytometer. **(a)** Distribution of cell sizes; **(b)** fluorescence with fluorochrome 1; **(c)** fluorescence with fluorochrome 2; and **(d)** granularity of cells (90° scatter).

procedures necessary to extract nuclei [14]. This may make significant differences to the levels of oncoproteins detected in the tumors and makes quantitative analysis difficult on preserved tissue.

All the techniques described in this section have been used to study oncogenes and tumor suppressor genes; the ways in which they may affect diagnosis, prognosis and therapy are described in the next two chapters.

## References

1. Sambrook, J., Fritsch, E.F. and Maniatis, T. (1989) *Molecular Cloning: A Laboratory Manual.* Cold Spring Harbor Laboratory Press, Cold Spring Harbor.
2. Berger, S.L. and Kimmel, A.R. (1987) *Methods in Enzymology,* Vol. 152. *Guide to Molecular Cloning Techniques.* Academic Press, New York.
3. Ehrlich, H.A. (1989) *Polymerase Chain Reaction Technology.* Stockton Press, New York.
4. Bos, J.L., Fearon, E.R., Hamilton, S.R., Verlaan-de Vries, M., van Boom, J.H., van der Eb, A.J. and Vogelstein, B. (1987) *Nature, 327,* 293.
5. Buckle, V.J and Craig, I. (1986) in *Human Genetic Diseases: a Practical Approach.* (K. Davies, ed.). IRL Press, Oxford, p. 85.
6. Tanaka, T., Slamon, D.J. and Cline, M.J. (1985) *Proc. Natl Acad. Sci. U.S.A., 82,* 3400.
7. Clark, R., Wong, G., Arnheim, N., Nitecki, D. and McCormick, F. (1985) *Proc. Natl Acad. Sci. U.S.A, 82,* 5280.
8. Horan Hand, P., Thor, A., Wunderlich, D., Muraro, R., Caruso, A. and Schlom, J. (1984) *Proc. Natl Acad. Sci. U.S.A., 81,* 5227.
9. Evan, G., Lewis, C.K., Ramsey, G. and Bishop, J.M. (1985) *Mol. Cell Biol., 5,* 3610.
10. Roth, J.A., Scuderi, P., Westin, E. and Gallo, R.C. (1985) *Surgery, 96,* 264.
11. Burnette, W.N. (1981) *Anal. Biochem., 112,* 195.
12. Young, B.D. (1986) in *Human Genetic Diseases: a Practical Approach* (K. Davies, ed.) IRL Press, Oxford, p. 101.
13. Stewart, C.C. (1989) *Arch. Pathol. Lab. Med., 113,* 634.
14. Lincoln, S.T. and Bauer, K.D. (1989) *Cytometry, 10,* 456.

# 4
# DIAGNOSTIC AND PROGNOSTIC APPLICATIONS OF ONCOGENES

Over the last decade, molecular techniques have been used to identify both oncogenes and tumor suppressor genes involved in the development of cancers. The primary aim of these studies is to use knowledge of the expression of these genes to benefit the patient, either for early diagnosis of tumors, as prognostic indicators, or eventually, as potential targets for therapy. The role of tumor suppressor genes is discussed in the next chapter, but here the value of oncogenes as diagnostic or prognostic markers will be considered.

The problem at the present time is to define a clear role for oncogenes in tumorigenesis. In the initial stages of research in this area, many different types of tumors were investigated for the presence of activated proto-oncogenes, and many were found. However, the numbers of tumors examined in individual studies were small. In many cases the analyses included cell lines derived from the original tumor and passaged many times *in vitro* . This has the potential for inducing further alterations in genes in addition to those seen in the tumor at the time of removal from the patient. Subsequently, larger studies have been carried out but the research is still in its infancy as it has not been possible to follow-up patients over an extended period of time. Several points are nevertheless clear. First, there is no absolute association between any one oncogene and any one type of tumor. Secondly, there is no clear evidence for the preferential activation of any oncogene at either early or late stages of tumor development as initially thought. Finally, there is no consistent evidence that expression of any one oncogene correlates with either good or poor prognosis. Amplification of *MYC* may correlate with poor prognosis in one type of tumor but with good prognosis in another.

A further problem in evaluating the potential of a particular oncogene is the contradictory nature of the results. For every study suggesting that expression of a particular oncogene indicates good prognosis, there is often one which states the reverse or which found no correlation between expression and any clinical criteria. There are some consistent results, for example, *MYCN* amplification has always correlated with rapid tumor progression in neuroblastomas, and *BCR–ABL* has a clear role in the development of CML and can be used diagnostically and prognostically for this disease.

In this chapter, the most important oncogenes identified in some of the more common tumors are discussed. Some of the less common tumors where specific roles have been assigned to a particular oncogene are also considered. The coverage is by no means complete but will hopefully indicate the potential for exploiting these genes in patient management. As the number of individual studies is very large, on the whole only major reviews covering these areas are referred to, but specific references are given if they describe a technique not covered elsewhere in this book.

## 4.1 Tumors of the gastro-intestinal tract

### 4.1.1 Colorectal cancer

Colorectal cancer is one of the most common of all human malignancies. The disease has long been known to develop in stages from adenomatous polyps to adenocarcinomas. Despite this knowledge, surgical treatment of the disease has had little impact on mortality in the last 20 years because patients rarely present with symptoms until late in the development of the disease. Alternative markers providing early detection would therefore be extremely valuable.

Screening for colorectal cancer by testing for fecal occult blood is possible, although the logistics of such a test are problematical. The test also has a high false negative rate and compliance is not always good. Many tumor-associated antigens such as carcino-embryonic antigen have been examined in colorectal cancer, but these markers are frequently of low specificity for the disease. Studies of the inherited form of colorectal cancer – FAP – have identified one defective gene involved in tumorigenesis (see Chapters 2 and 5). Several oncogenes have also been identified in colorectal cancer and some have a prognostic role in the disease. A pattern of successive genetic changes as the disease progresses is now becoming apparent (see Section 2.5.1).

Early studies of colorectal cancer using cell lines revealed amplification of *MYC* and *MYB* but the lines used probably represented atypical cases. Subsequently, no major role has been identified for either amplification or rearrangement of any oncogene in colorectal cancer [1].

Increased levels of *MYC* transcripts have been detected by Northern blotting in up to 70% of colorectal cancers, but have not correlated with disease progression, histological diagnosis or Dukes staging [1].

Immunohistochemical studies with the monoclonal antibodies Myc1-6E10 and Myc1-9E10 have confirmed the Northern blotting results by showing high levels of the *MYC* protein, p62, in colorectal cancers (*Figure 4.1*). Some studies have found a correlation with tumor differentiation but others found no difference. In addition, increased levels of p62 have also been associated with inflammatory conditions such as Crohn's disease and ulcerative colitis. Some uncertainty has arisen in the literature concerning the use of Myc1-6E10 because it appears to recognize a protein present in both the nucleus and the cytoplasm. Suggestions for this unexpected distribution of p62 have included

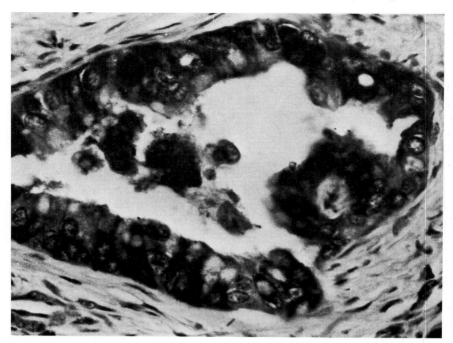

**Figure 4.1**: *p62 expression in the cytoplasm of cells from a colorectal cancer as detected by Myc1-6E10.*

poor tissue fixation conditions or extraction of p62 by salt and/or low temperatures. Alternatively, it is possible that the antibody cross-reacts with an unrelated antigen. A review of the staining patterns seen with this antibody in colorectal cancer has suggested that the observed expression is largely a function of the fixation process; the protein recognized is probably p62, but the possibility of non-specific binding has not been totally excluded [1].

Studies of the RNA and protein levels confirm that high levels of *MYC* expression are to be found in colorectal tumors, probably because the oncogene is a marker of cell proliferation. Whether deregulation and high expression of *MYC* are required to maintain the tumorigenic state has yet to be determined. With two exceptions, there have been very few diagnostic or prognostic implications of *MYC* expression levels in colorectal cancers.

One recent study has suggested a role for *MYC* as a marker for monitoring the transition from the benign to malignant state. Levels of *MYC* transcripts determined by Northern blotting were closely related to histological type and size of colorectal polyps. In particular, adenomas containing carcinoma *in situ* or high-grade dysplasia expressed high levels of *MYC*. This study was small, however, so its findings still require confirmation [2].

Elevated expression of the *MYC* gene has also been particularly associated with tumors on the distal part of the colon. On the basis of this observation it has been suggested that elevated levels of *MYC* are a marker of those sporadic colorectal cancers which correspond to the inherited carcinoma developing in FAP and involving the *APC* gene. Additional studies following this observation have indicated loss of *MYC* regulation in carcinomas defective in the chromosomal region containing the *APC* gene. These results are consistent with the possibility that the product of the *APC* gene exerts its effect by deregulating *MYC* [3].

Alterations in *RAS* have been studied extensively in colorectal cancer. There has been no evidence for amplification or rearrangement of the gene, but elevated expression of *RAS* and frequent mutations in both *KRAS* and *HRAS* have been identified.

One study demonstrated elevated levels of the *RAS* gene family transcripts in both premalignant and malignant tumors of the colon and rectum, suggesting that elevated expression might be critical in the process of carcinogenesis. As all polyps do not progress, despite showing increased *RAS* expression, the observation is consistent with the involvement of other genes in the development of cancers. In contrast, a second study found elevated *KRAS* and *HRAS* in only a small percentage of carcinomas and increased levels of *KRAS* in only one polyp. There was a correlation between poor prognosis and elevated levels of *KRAS* and *HRAS* if increased levels of *FOS* and *MYC* transcripts were also present in the same tumor. As both studies were small it is difficult to determine the significance of these observations [1].

Many immunohistochemical studies have used the Y13 259 or RAP 5 antibodies to investigate *RAS* expression, with variable results. In some studies Y13 259 has been found to react with tissues at all stages of colon carcinogenesis, but others have found that it reacts most intensely with adenomas, suggesting that increased expression is a relatively early event. Immunoblotting studies showed that the antibody reacted primarily with extracts of Dukes stage B and C tumors, rarely with Dukes D and never with colorectal metastases. Preliminary studies with RAP 5 suggested that elevated expression of *RAS* was a relatively late event in carcinogenesis because reactivity was seen primarily in carcinomas and not in adenomatous polyps. More recently, studies with RAP 5 have consistently shown the most enhanced reactivity with early epithelial dysplastic lesions and carcinoma *in situ*, a result confirmed with a second antibody [4]. Overall, enhanced expression of *RAS* p21, whether measured immunohistochemically or by increased transcript level, appears to be an early event in colon carcinogenesis. There is little correlation of *RAS* expression with histological classification of tumors, with depth of invasion or with stage of disease [1].

Analysis of point mutations in the *RAS* gene has provided more consistent results, suggesting that *RAS* mutations occur early in the development of colorectal tumors. The use of the PCR has allowed the selective amplification of specific sequences and has undoubtedly contributed to the reliability of the analysis. As small amounts of DNA can be analyzed it has been possible to select the areas of tissue to be used carefully, by extracting the DNA from tumor-rich regions of histological specimens without including areas of inflammatory or normal cells [5]. Using these techniques, over 40% of colorectal tumors have been found to have an activated *RAS* gene, the majority of the mutations occurring in codon 12 of *KRAS* [6].

Confirmation that mutations in *RAS* are an early event came from the finding that a high proportion of *RAS* mutations occur in adenomas, in tumors originating in adenomas and in both the benign and malignant areas of the same tumor. The mutational event appears to occur before the tumor becomes aneuploid [1]. A large study has investigated the timing of these events in colorectal cancer in relation to other genetic alterations. In addition to 50% of carcinomas, 50% of large adenomas contain a *RAS* gene mutation but the mutation has been found in only 9% of those adenomas < 1 cm in size. There are two possibilities for these observations. Either the mutation is the initiating event occurring in a subset of tumors which are the ones that progress, or the mutation may be a progressive event occurring in one cell of an existing small adenoma causing it to develop into a large one [6]. As already discussed in Section 2.5.1, an accumulation of other events occur following the *RAS* mutation. All or some of these are necessary before a colorectal tumor can develop.

There is no diagnostic value to the presence of *RAS* mutations in colorectal tumors at the present time. However, the use of the PCR to identify mutations in the gene may aid detection of early stage disease in the near future. The presence of subsequent cumulative changes may also be of prognostic value in patients with colorectal cancer.

### 4.1.2 Stomach cancer

Although there has been an overall decrease in the mortality rates in gastric cancer, it is still a major cause of all cancer deaths. With the advent of screening programs, particularly endoscopic examination, there has been an increase in the detection of early disease. Tumors are commonly classified, on the basis of the Lauren classification, into intestinal or diffuse types. Unlike colorectal cancer there is no clearly defined premalignant lesion, although intestinal metaplasia, particularly type-3 disease, is frequently associated with cancers, especially the intestinal type. In addition, high-grade dysplasia has been considered to precede gastric carcinoma. A marker which could help to identify premalignant lesions and also a marker for prognosis might help to reduce the mortality from this disease.

*MYC* amplification has occasionally been found in stomach cancers. In five out of 27 samples of gastric carcinomas, one study found evidence of *MYC* amplification of up to 30-fold, but all tumors examined had been passaged and maintained in nude mice. In one isolated case of a squamous cell cancer of the stomach, there was evidence for co-amplification of *MYC* and *ERBB1*.

In gastric cancers, studies of *MYC* gene expression using the monoclonal antibody Myc1-6E10 found elevated levels of the protein in approximately 40% of cases (*Figure 4.2*), but there was no correlation between stage of disease, histological classification or differentiation. Increased expression was also seen in inflammatory lesions in the stomach, including metaplastic and dysplastic lesions (*Figure 4.2*), but as in the colon this probably correlates with *MYC* as a marker of the hyperproliferative state [1]. The antibody has been observed to react with a population of cells on the tip of the interfoveolar crests of the gastric mucosa, which are distinct from the normal foveolar cells or regenerative epithelial cells (*Figure 4.2*). They have been proposed to be a

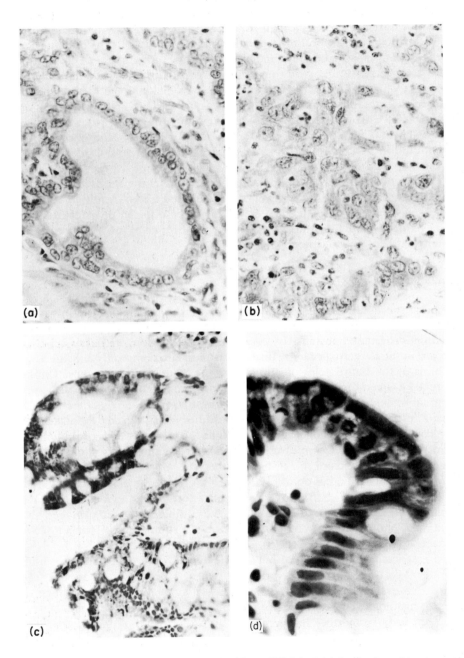

***Figure 4.2:*** *p62 expression detected by Myc1-6E10 in (**a**) intestinal gastric cancer, (**b**) diffuse type of gastric cancer, (**c**) intestinal metaplasia, and (**d**) tip lesion.*

precursor of type-3 intestinal metaplasia and there may be a link between this type of metaplasia and the intestinal variant of gastric cancer, but this hypothesis still requires confirmation [7]. Again, the possibility of antibody cross-reactivity may mean that the target is not p62. The overall results of *MYC* expression suggest little prognostic or diagnostic role for *MYC* in gastric carcinomas.

The expression of the epidermal growth factor (EGF) receptor has been shown to play a role in the biological behavior of some tumors. In immuno-histochemical studies, between 20 and 50% of gastric cancers have been shown to express EGFR. Preliminary studies showed no correlation with histological differentiation or presence of lymph-node metastases, but in a much larger study of over 200 patients the incidence of EGFRs was significantly higher in well-differentiated tumors. The study also demonstrated that the EGFR was a marker of highly malignant tumors, conferring a much worse prognosis [8].

There has been little evidence in any study for expression of *RAS* p21 in benign lesions, either immunohistochemically or by radioimmunoassay. Enhanced expression of *RAS* p21 has been detected immunohistochemically in over 60% of gastric cancers using RAP 5 antibody, with higher levels of *RAS* p21 in advanced cancers. Patients with stage III or IV disease who express *HRAS* have been shown to have a worse prognosis than those whose tumors were negative. Elevated levels of transforming growth factor alpha (TGF-α) together with *HRAS* in gastric cancer have been correlated with a significantly worse prognosis. Overall, the data suggest that in stomach cancer increased *RAS* expression may be important in progression rather than being involved at an early stage as seen in colorectal cancers.

## 4.2 Lung tumors

Lung cancers are divided into small cell lung cancers (SCLCs) and non-small cell lung cancers (N-SCLCs). The latter are further subdivided into adenocarcinomas, squamous cell carcinomas and large cell carcinomas. SCLCs show the worst prognosis. As with colorectal and gastric cancers, there has been little improvement in survival rates in lung cancer over the past 30 years.

Abnormal expression of all three members of the *MYC* family (*MYCN*, *MYCL* and *MYC*) has been detected in lung cancers. Amplification of one or other of the *MYC* genes is found in 10–20% of lung tumors. The tumors of SCLC patients with amplification of *MYC* have been shown to be the more aggressive and these patients have consequently had a significantly worse prognosis [9].

Increased *MYCN* expression in SCLC detected by *in-situ* hybridization has also been correlated with poor response to chemotherapy, rapid tumor growth and short survival times [9]. Elevated *MYC* expression has also been demonstrated in 19% of SCLCs and 42% of N-SCLCs using the Myc1-9E10 antibody, but no correlation between elevated expression and survival could be shown in these patients [9].

As survival from metastatic lung cancer is so poor, enhancers of chemotherapy have been sought. As a preliminary to targeted therapy with antibodies, the ability of the monoclonal antibody Myc1-6E10 to localize lung

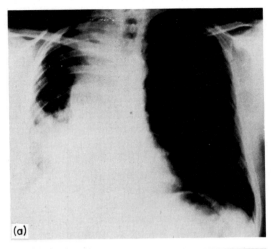

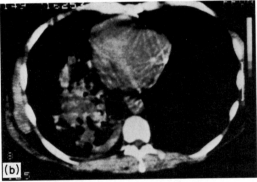

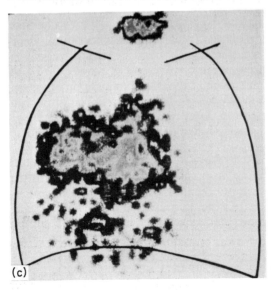

**Figure 4.3:** *(a) X-ray showing primary tumor in right lung and mediastinal metastases, (b) CT scan, and (c) image of lung tumor following localization of $^{131}$I-labeled antibody to p62. Figure reproduced from [10] with permission from the* British Journal of Cancer.

tumors was investigated. Following radiolabeling with $^{131}$I, this antibo
administered intraveneously to 20 patients with malignant disease. G
camera imaging 24 and 48 h later showed good tumor localization in 12 out of
14 patients with primary bronchial carcinoma (*Figure 4.3*). In the remaining
six patients who had pulmonary metastases from a variety of tumors, no localization was found. As the p62 protein is located primarily in the cell nucleus,
the localization was presumed to depend on release of nuclear contents following cell death [10]. Although this protein is not the ideal target for such
studies, it was the first to show the feasibility of this approach to targeted
therapy (see Chapter 6).

Increased expression of the *RAS* gene has been detected in lung cancers,
as have structural abnormalities in the gene. Differential expression of *RAS*
p21 determined by Western blotting with Y13 259 has been correlated with
histological classification. In one study, 82% of squamous cell cancers had increased levels of p21 whereas only 8% of non-squamous cell tumors showed
any increase in expression, thus correlating increased expression with histological classification [1].

The PCR has been used to identify point mutations in *KRAS* in N-SCLCs,
primarily in adenocarcinomas. This study suggested that carcinogens in
tobacco smoke were the cause of the mutations as there was a strong correlation between the incidence of mutations and the smoking habits of patients.
Primary N-SCLCs with *KRAS* mutations have been shown to be smaller and
to have a lower metastatic potential than tumors without *RAS* mutations. If
the presence of *KRAS* mutations can be confirmed as a good prognostic indicator it may of use in planning chemotherapy for certain patients [9].

Finally, RFLPs associated with *HRAS* have been shown to be possible
genetic markers for lung cancer. Four common alleles are identified in the
population along with a number of rarer alleles. An abnormal allele distribution has been associated with the more aggressive N-SCLCs compared with
normal cells or SCLCs, suggesting a degree of genetic predisposition to this
disease [11]. A similar RFLP has been associated with *MYCL* and one
particular allele has been associated with metastatic disease.

High levels of EGFRs have been associated with N-SCLC, particularly
squamous carcinomas. The strongest staining with an anti-EGFR antibody
was associated with stage-III tumors, suggesting, as with other tumor types,
that expression of the EGFR may be associated with growth and metastasis.
An antibody to the external domain of the receptor may prove to be better for
targeting purposes than the antibody to p62 for the localization of lung
tumors. High concentrations of the EGFR in these tumors with poor prognosis also suggests a possible target for therapy [12].

## 4.3 Breast cancer

Breast cancer is the cause of death in 20% of all females who die from cancer,
and survival figures have not altered significantly over the years. The tumors
are classified as non-invasive or invasive, the majority (76%) belonging to the
group of invasive ductal breast cancers. Patients can be staged using the
clinical characteristics of tumor diameter (T), lymph node involvement (N)
and the presence of distant metastases (M), hence the nomenclature TNM

staging. Prognostic factors include lymph node status, degree of differentiation of the tumor and the presence of estrogen and/or progesterone receptors. The DNA content (ploidy) of tumors has been suggested as a prognostic indicator but its use is limited at present.

Breast cancers have probably been studied more than any other tumor type with regard to oncogene expression. Either *MYC*, *ERBB2* or one of the *RAS* family have been found to be expressed in over 60% of samples.

Very few examples of rearrangements or amplifications of the *MYCN* or *MYCL* genes have been found in breast cancer. On the other hand, there is considerable evidence for *MYC* amplification although the incidence varies from one study to another (6–57%). Three large studies of *MYC* amplification in breast cancer have produced different conclusions as to the value of this marker in prognosis [1].

In one study, including 80 primary breast carcinomas as well as benign tissues and nodal metastases, amplification was the major alteration in the *MYC* gene occurring in 18% of tumors, and one example of a rearrangment was also seen. Amplification was primarily associated with infiltrating ductal carcinomas and poorly differentiated tumors. No stage-I tumors showed any abnormalities in *MYC*. A significant correlation was seen between amplification of *MYC* and poor short-term prognosis, implicating this gene in the progression of breast cancer. In a second study of tumors from 121 patients, over 30% had abnormalities in *MYC*. There was a significant correlation between tumors of post-menopausal patients and amplification of *MYC*, but no correlation with tumor grade, receptor status or presence of metastatic disease was found. No survival rates were presented in this study. Finally, a prospective study of 125 patients found amplification of *MYC* in 18% of cases but no clinical correlations were detected, except a highly significant association between *MYC* amplification and inflammatory carcinomas, suggesting that *MYC* might contribute to the rapid progression of this subtype of breast cancer.

Increased levels of *MYC* mRNA have also been found in breast cancer and have not always correlated with gene amplification. In one study almost 50% of tumors had elevated mRNA levels and this correlated with the presence of lymph node metastases. Amplification was seen in only 11% of tumors [1].

Monoclonal antibodies Myc1-6E10 and Myc1-9E10 have both been used to study p62 levels in breast cancers but have not clarified the role of *MYC* in this disease. Seventy per cent of cases in one study, using monoclonal antibody Myc1-9E10, showed expression of p62 in both the nucleus and occasionally in the cytoplasm, but there was no correlation with histopathological grade, presence of metastases in the lymph nodes, or receptor status [1]. This antibody may not be of value for detecting abnormalities in the *MYC* gene, because discrepancies have been demonstrated between the levels of *MYC* protein, as determined immunohistochemically, and the levels of mRNA measured by *in-situ* hybridization. Neither of these techniques could be used to indicate the presence of amplification [13]. These results suggest that there may be problems in using measurement of oncoprotein levels with monoclonal antibodies in routinely processed tissues as a measure of abnormalities in the oncogene itself.

Finally, a sensitive enzyme assay has been used as a means of measuring *MYC* oncoprotein expression in tissue extracts. All tumors had elevated levels of p62 compared with normal tissue, but no correlation with age, nodal status, receptor status, histopathological grade or survival was observed. There was, however, an association between tumor size (T) and high levels of *MYC* oncoprotein expression [1].

Taken together these results do not show any clearly defined diagnostic or prognostic role for *MYC* in breast cancer. Any role it does have is likely to be complex. More useful information has been obtained from measurements of *ERBB2* and the *RAS* gene family.

The majority of studies have detected elevated levels of *HRAS* mRNA in primary breast carcinomas. Elevated expression was associated with advanced histological types. In contrast, a further study detected elevated expression of *NRAS* and *KRAS*, but only one tumor showed any increase in *HRAS* [1].

Increased expression of *RAS* p21 has been detected in 63–83% of malignant breast tumors compared with low levels in benign tissues. A single study was unable to detect differences in *RAS* p21 expression between malignant and benign breast tumors. In general there are no significant clinical correlations, although one study demonstrated higher *RAS* p21 expression in carcinomas from post-menopausal women. A direct-binding quantitative competition radioimmunoassay has been developed for *RAS* p21 using monoclonal antibody Y13 259 to determine absolute levels of the protein. Again, approximately two-thirds of carcinomas demonstrate high levels of the protein compared with lactating breast and benign tissues. Recent studies using this technique demonstrated higher levels of p21 in post-menopausal patients. Levels of *RAS* p21 have also been determined in breast tissue using Western blotting techniques and the results have confirmed the immunohistochemical findings of high levels of the protein in malignant tissues. An association was also found between high levels of *RAS* p21 and extent of tumor and a significant correlation was seen between high levels and short disease-free interval.

Studies of the *RAS* family in breast cancer have therefore found little evidence for point mutations or structural alterations in the genes, but high levels of *RAS* appear to be associated with progression of breast cancer and poor prognosis [1].

As in lung cancer, polymorphisms associated with *HRAS* have been investigated in breast cancer. In one study, four common alleles and 16 rare alleles were found in the normal and cancer-bearing populations. The frequency of two particular common alleles was diminished in the breast cancer patients with concomitant increases in two rare alleles. One of these rare alleles was significantly associated with breast cancer and is potentially of use in risk analysis. In a second study, *HRAS* allele loss has been found in breast tumors and correlates significantly with grade-III tumors, lack of estrogen/progesterone receptors and the presence of distant metastases. A third study has confirmed that allele loss correlates with low levels of estrogen receptors [1].

*ERBB2* amplification in breast cancer has been demonstrated by many investigators, in frequencies ranging from 10 to 30%. In a preliminary study, amplification of *ERBB2* correlated with poor prognosis in lymph-node positive patients. Several subsequent studies confirmed this finding, but others have been unable to show any correlation. The workers who produced the initial results have corroborated their findings in a large study of 526 patients [14] and two other groups have found similar results in lymph-node negative breast cancer. In one study co-amplification of *ERBB2* and *ERBA* has been found in 23% of breast tumors and has been shown to be a stong indicator of metastatic potential.

Antibodies to the *ERBB2* protein have also been used to study over-expression of *ERBB2* in breast cancer and there are several reports which correlate the levels of *ERBB2* protein with gene amplification. As with direct analysis of gene amplification, immunostaining for *ERBB2* protein as a prognostic marker has shown both positive and negative correlations. Strong staining was found in 9, 14 and 17% of cases of breast cancer in three different studies. Several groups found no relationship between staining and stage, node status, receptor status or size of tumor, but others have shown a significant association between reactivity and mortality or recurrence [15]. A recent study has correlated *ERBB2* over-expression with the presence of hematogenous metastases.

These conflicting results are likely to be due to variations in the numbers of patients examined, differences in antibodies used, length of follow-up and methods of scoring immunoreactivity. The immunohistochemical technique has potential as a routine method for the analysis of expression of *ERBB2* in tumors, once all the parameters have been carefully evaluated and standardized. Data obtained from such studies should confirm or refute a role for *ERBB2* as a prognostic indicator in this disease.

## 4.4 Neuroblastoma

*MYCN* was one of the first oncogenes demonstrated to be of clinical significance and in contrast to many of the findings discussed above, the association is not controversial. *MYCN* was initially identified because of a strong association between DMs or HSRs and human neuroblastomas. These regions were shown to contain a DNA sequence which showed partial homology with the *MYC* gene. Both neuroblastoma cell lines and tumors were shown to carry amplified *MYCN*. Subsequently, similar results were found in other tumors derived from the neuroectoderm, such as SCLC and retinoblastoma. Experimental systems have been used to demonstrate that high expression of *MYCN* can modulate cell growth.

Stage III and IV neuroblastomas have a poor prognosis, with only 10–30% survival at 2 years. A strong correlation has been found between stage III and IV disease and *MYCN* amplification. In contrast, stage IV-s tumors which frequently regress have rarely been associated with *MYCN* amplification [16]. *In-situ* hybridization has been used to detect increased levels of *MYCN* mRNA and correlates well with determination of gene copy number. This technique can be used to detect increased expression of *MYCN* in a largely negative cell population where direct analysis of amplification would give a negative result.

Tumors from occasional patients have shown no evidence of *MYCN* amplification but have still had a poor prognosis, suggesting that the correlation is not perfect. Loss of the short arm of chromosome 1 has also been detected in neuroblastomas and shown to be independent of *MYCN* amplification. Therefore, as with all the other tumors, it seems that more than one gene is involved in the tumorigenesis of neuroblastoma.

Although medulloblastoma shares many features in common with neuroblastoma, no evidence of *MYCN* amplification has been detected in these tumors. Instead, over-expression of the gene has been found in approximately 50% of tumors and has been shown to correlate with shorter disease-free survival.

## 4.5 Genito-urinary tumors

### 4.5.1 Ovarian cancer

There are several similarities between ovarian and breast cancers, for example, both often express steroid hormone receptors and it is suggested that they have common etiological factors. Several prognostic factors have been identified in ovarian cancer, including stage of disease, presence or absence of ascites and volume of residual disease following surgery. Histological grading and ploidy are also strongly associated with clinical outcome.

Amplification of *MYC* has been detected in ovarian cancer cell lines and in single cases of ovarian cancer. Immunostaining with the antibody Myc1-6E10, showed that all malignant mucinous ovarian cancers expressed high levels of p62. The least differentiated tumors expressed the lowest levels of p62, which is in keeping with expression in colonic, testicular and the majority of reports of breast cancers, confirming a potential role for *MYC* in cellular differentiation.

Amplification of *KRAS* has been found only occasionally in ovarian cancers but does not appear to play a fundamental role in tumor development or progression. The *RAS* p21 protein has also been detected in advanced ovarian cancers using RAP 5, but no correlation with histological type, grade, ploidy or clinical outcome could be demonstrated.

Like breast cancers, approximately 30% of ovarian cancers carry amplified *ERBB2*, but here the presence of the amplified oncogene appears to correlate with poor survival. In one study, the survival times for patients with one, two to five, or over 10 copies of *ERBB2* were 1879, 959 and 243 days, respectively.

### 4.5.2 Cervical cancers

A number of prognostic factors have been linked to the progression of cervical cancers, including depth of stromal invasion, lesion depth and nodal involvement. In particular, human papilloma virus (HPV) has been found to be integrated into malignant cells and the presence of the virus (in specific subtypes) in pre-malignant lesions indicates a poor prognosis. Abnormal expression of several oncogenes also has prognostic value.

Amplification and over-expression of *MYC* has been shown to be more frequent in advanced tumors of the uterine cervix compared with early tumors. In tumor samples of 72 untreated patients with carcinoma of the cervix, over-expression was detected in 35% of cases. This over-expression was not a consequence of amplification which was seen in only 8% of cases. There was no relationship between *MYC* over-expression and stage, nodal status or age. However, there was an eightfold greater risk of relapse for patients with over-expression of *MYC*, which outweighed even nodal status as a prognostic factor [1].

Elevated expression of *RAS* p21, as demonstrated by the use of antibody Y13 259, has been found in malignant as opposed to benign or premalignant lesions. In the small cell type of squamous cell carcinomas, tumors with elevated expression of *RAS* p21 were shown to have a better prognosis than negative tumors. Expression of *RAS* p21 together with histological type may therefore be of prognostic significance in carcinomas of the cervix in specific histological types [1].

Mutations at codon 12 of the *HRAS* gene have also been found in cervical cancer and in one study were correlated with poor prognosis [1].

### 4.5.3 Testicular cancer

Strong expression of p62 has been detected in differentiating areas of testicular tumors. In a flow-cytometric study of p62 expression in nuclei extracted from paraffin blocks, increasing levels of p62 correlated with increasing differentiation of teratomas. Patients who had no recurrence 3 years after diagnosis showed a significantly higher level of p62 than those who developed a recurrence in this time period. Expression of *MYC* may therefore prove to be of prognostic significance in this disease [17].

### 4.5.4 Renal cell cancer

The clinical behaviour of this disease is unpredictable, although a few features, such as stage of tumor and ploidy, are partially correlated with prognosis. The disease is highly metastatic, with 30% of patients having metastases at the time of diagnosis.

A study of *MYCL* RFLPs in patients with renal cell cancer has shown no significant differences between the RFLP patterns of normal and tumor DNA. However, the presence of metastases was associated with lack of a particular allele suggesting that this RFLP may be a marker of genetic predisposition to the formation of metastases rather than the development of primary disease.

### 4.5.5 Prostatic cancer

This disease also has an extremely variable natural history, ranging from a non-invasive disease to a rapidly metastatic disease which is fatal within a short time following diagnosis. It is frequently diagnosed incidentally at the time of surgery during transurethral resection for urinary obstruction. Although factors such as histological grade have been evaluated as prognostic factors, there is considerable uncertainty concerning their use. Tumor markers such as carcino-embryonic antigen and prostatic acid phosphatase have not proven to be consistently useful.

Levels of *MYC* have been determined in prostate cancer and benign prostatic hyperplasia to determine whether the level of expression of the gene can distinguish between malignant and benign disease or can predict aggressive disease. Significantly higher levels of *MYC* expression have been found in malignant disease and a subset of patients had increased levels compared with the rest of the cancer group. At present the prognostic value of these findings remains to be determined.

Expression of *RAS* p21 has been examined in prostate cancer using RAP 5. Staining was particularly associated with high grade, and presumably more metastatic, tumors. In a semi-quantitative assay, there was a significant association between degree of nuclear aplasia and expression of *RAS* p21. Compared with the tumor markers carcino-embryonic antigen and prostate-specific antigen, *RAS* p21 was the only phenotypic marker which correlated with tumor grade.

## 4.6 Hematological malignancies

Many oncogenes have been identified in leukemias and lymphomas because of the presence of consistent chromosomal translocations which can be identified cytogenetically. The breakpoint in one of the chromosomes has frequently been shown to occur in, or close to, an oncogene (*Table 4.1*). In addition, other oncogenes commonly identified in human tumors, such as the *RAS* family, have also been found associated with hematological malignancies. A few common examples of the diagnostic and prognostic value of oncogenes follow.

**Table 4.1**: *Chromosomal translocations in leukemias and lymphomas associated with oncogenes*

| Disease | Translocation | Oncogene |
|---|---|---|
| B-CLL | t(11;14) | *BCL1* |
| Burkitt's lymphoma | t(8;14) | *MYC* |
| | t(2;8) | |
| | t(8;22) | |
| CML (AML and ALL) | t(9;22) | *ABL* |
| Follicular lymphoma | t(14;18) | *BCL2* |

### 4.6.1 MYC *in hematological malignancy*

The involvement of the *MYC* gene in Burkitt's lymphoma is probably one of the most studied of all events involving oncogenes. The translocation between chromosomes 8 and 14 is a highly consistent and specific rearrangment found in 75–85% of Burkitt's lymphoma patients. In the remaining 15–25% of patients the translocation occurs between chromosomes 8 and either 2 or 22. This translocation places the *MYC* gene from chromosome 8 next to the immunoglobulin heavy chain locus on chromosome 14 or the κ and λ constant regions, on chromosomes 2 and 22, 3′ of the *MYC* gene on chromosome 8

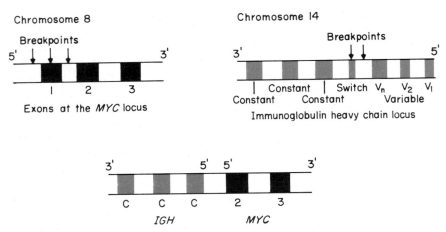

**Figure 4.4:** *Molecular basis of the translocation between the* MYC *gene on chromosome 8 and the immunoglobulin heavy chain on chromosome 14 which occurs in the majority of cases of Burkitt's lymphoma.*

(*Figure 4.4* and *Figure 1.9*). In the commonest translocation the breakpoint on chromosome 8 occurs on the 5' side of the second exon of the *MYC* gene. This means that the two coding exons of the gene – exons 2 and 3 – are always translocated and placed close to the constant region of the immunoglobulin heavy chain locus on chromosome 14. In the two less common translocations the breakpoint is distal to the *MYC* gene. In all cases, the coding exons of *MYC* do not undergo any structural rearrangement. Instead the translocation results in deregulation of *MYC*. Following the general rule that the development of malignancy is a multistage event, other changes are necessary for the development of Burkitt's lymphoma. In one model the first change is chronic stimulation and activation of the B cells by infectious agents, primarily Epstein–Barr virus, leading to the emergence of immortalized clones. The second stage is the translocation involving *MYC*. A second model proposes that these two events occur in the reverse order. Additional changes in other oncogenes are likely to follow these two steps [18].

A study of increased *MYC* expression in other malignant lymphomas, using the antibody Myc1-6E10, did not show any significant association, although T-cell immunoblastic malignant lymphomas were consistently positively stained. Flow-cytometric detection of p62 has demonstrated a correlation between *MYC* protein levels and the aggressiveness of malignant non-Hodgkins lymphomas of B-cell origin.

Preliminary evidence has suggested that there is variation in an RFLP associated with the *MYCL* locus, which plays a role in both survival and susceptibility to non-Hodgkins lymphoma and acute lymphoblastic lymphoma.

### 4.6.2 RAS family in hematological malignancy

Altered *RAS* genes have been associated with a number of hematological malignancies. In myelodysplastic syndrome (MDS) and acute myeloid leukemia (AML), a mutation has been found in the *RAS* gene in approximately one-third of cases: this is usually in *NRAS*, occasionally in *KRAS* and infrequently in *HRAS*. Several studies have suggested that patients with MDS and a *RAS* mutation are more likely to progress to AML and hence have the worst prognosis. However, as there are examples of MDS patients with a *RAS* mutation in their multipotent stem cells who have stable disease, this marker is unlikely to be of use on its own as a prognostic indicator. Secondly, AML patients with or without *RAS* mutations do not have a significantly different prognosis. Alternative roles for the *RAS* mutation may be as a marker for monitoring the effects of chemotherapy or detecting minimal residual disease [19].

In a large study of childhood ALL, point mutations were found in 6% of cases at codons 12 or 13 of *NRAS*. These cases had a significantly higher risk of hematological relapse and a trend towards a lower rate of complete remission than those without *RAS* mutations. Presence of *RAS* mutations was independent of other high-risk factors for ALL and may therefore be a useful prognostic indicator.

### 4.6.3 BCL2 *in follicular lymphomas*

A translocation between chromosomes 14 and 18 is consistently found in approximately 85% of follicular lymphomas and involves the putative oncogene *BCL2* on chromosome 18 placing it next to the immunoglobulin heavy chain locus.

Progression of follicular lymphomas to a more aggressive form is frequently associated with overgrowth of subclones containing chromosomal changes, in addition to the characteristic 14;18 translocation. In some cases this is associated with an 8;14 translocation involving the *MYC* gene, as seen in Burkitt's lymphoma.

### 4.6.4 ABL *in hematological malignancy*

A 9;22 translocation is found in approximately 90% of all cases of CML. It is not diagnostic for this disease, as it is also present in 25% of adult ALLs, in 2–10% of childhood ALLs and in occasional cases of AML. The breakpoint on chromosome 9 occurs on the 5′ side of the first coding exon of the *ABL* proto-oncogene. On chromosome 22, the breakpoint occurs within the *BCR* [or major cluster region (*MCR*), as it is now called]. This 5.8 kb DNA region contains four small exons and is part of the *PHL* gene. As a result of the translocation, a fusion gene is produced which, following splicing, is transcribed to give an 8.5 kb mRNA encoding a 210 kd fusion protein. This altered protein exhibits elevated constitutive protein-tyrosine kinase activity (*Figure 4.5*). Molecular analysis of ALL reveals a second class of rearrangement in some cases. Here, the breakpoint in the *PHL* gene occurs near the 5′ end, resulting in a 7 kb chimeric mRNA encoding a 190 kd protein which again has altered tyrosine kinase activity (*Figure 4.5*). The production of these fusion proteins is likely to be an important step in the pathogenesis of these diseases but it is still not clear whether the translocation is the primary event in tumorigenesis.

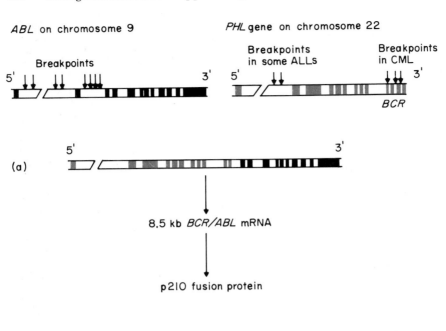

ABL on chromosome 9

PHL gene on chromosome 22

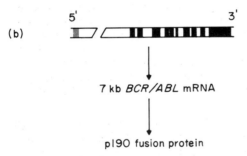

Figure 4.5: Molecular basis of the Ph[1] translocation seen in (a) CML and (b) some cases of ALL.

Although the Ph[1] chromosome can be detected cytogenetically, molecular techniques are now being used to aid diagnosis, and many cases previously thought to be Ph[1] negative have now been shown by Southern blotting to contain the rearrangement [20] (*Figure 4.6*). The accurate detection of this marker is important because patients who are Ph[1] negative generally show reduced survival rates. Molecular techniques have also been used to detect the presence or absence of specific *BCR* exons. It has recently been shown that the presence or absence of exon 3 of the *BCR* gene accounts for some of the variability in the disease duration, thereby influencing the timing of onset of blast crisis. Patients with Ph[1] chromosomes containing exon 3 have a statistically shorter disease duration and more rapid onset of blast crisis [21].

The ability to detect the presence of a *BCR/ABL* fusion gene by PCR has also allowed the development of a very sensitive diagnostic test for CML. In addition, it has been used successfully in the detection of the presence of residual disease following bone marrow transplantation. This might allow early therapy of patients with residual disease and sustain remission. The

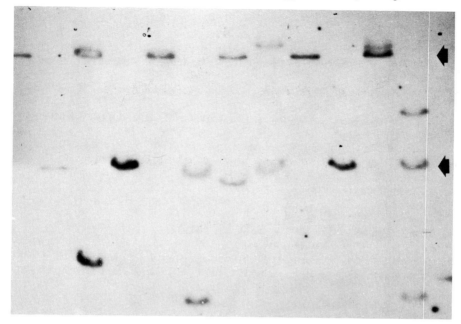

**Figure 4.6**: *Autoradiograph of DNA samples hybridized with probe BCR-G showing rearrangements in Ph¹-positive patients. Lanes 1 and 2 – negative controls; lanes 3 and 4, 5 and 6, 7 and 8, and 9 and 10 show DNA from four individuals with CML; and lanes 11 and 12 are known positive controls. For each pair of samples, DNA in the left-hand lane was digested with EcoRI and that in the right with HindIII. The positions of the normal bands are marked with an arrow. Autoradiograph courtesy of John Quick, North Trent Regional Molecular Genetics Service, Sheffield, U.K.*

major problem with this technique is also the reason for its use, that is, its high sensitivity. The persistence of low levels of Ph¹-positive cells has been a consistent finding and it is not yet clear how many of these cells are necessary to re-establish disease. In the near future long-term follow-up of these patients will hopefully clarify this point and allow post-transplant therapy to be initiated where necessary.

## References

1. Field, J.K. and Spandidos, D.A. (1990) *Anticancer Res.*, **10**, 1.
2. Imaseki, H., Hayashi, H., Taira, M., Ito, Y., Tabata, Y., Onada, S., Isono, K. and Tatibana, M. (1989) *Cancer*, **64**, 704.
3. Astrin, S.M. and Costanzi, C. (1989) *Seminars Oncology*, **16**, 138.
4. Jansson, D.S., Radosevich, J.A., Carney, W.P., Rosen, S.T., Schlom, J., Staren, E.D., Hyser, M.J. and Gould, V.E. (1990) *Cancer*, **65**, 1329.
5. Bos, J.L., Fearon, E.R., Hamilton, S.R., Verlaan-de Fries, M., van Boom, J.H., van der Eb, A.J. and Vogelstein, B. (1987) *Nature*, **327**, 293.
6. Fearon, E.R. and Vogelstein, B. (1990) *Cell*, **61**, 759.
7. Newbold, K.M., Macdonald, F. and Allum, W.H. (1988) *J. Pathol.*, **155**, 311.
8. Tahara, E., Sumiyoshi, H., Hata, J., Yasui, W., Taniyama, K., Hayashi, T., Nagae, S. and Sakamoto, S. (1986) *Jap. J. Cancer Res.*, **77**, 145.

9. Viallet, J. and Minna, J.D. (1990) *Am. J. Resp. Cell, Molec. Biol.*, **2**, 225.
10. Chan, S.Y.T., Evan, G.I., Titson, A., Watson, J., Wraight, P. and Sikora, K. (1986) *Br. J. Cancer*, **54**, 761.
11. Heighway, J., Thatcher, N., Cerny, T. and Hasleton, P.S. (1986) *Br. J. Cancer*, **53**, 453.
12. Veale, D., Ashcroft, T., Marsh, C., Gibson, G.J. and Harris, A.L. (1987) *Br. J. Cancer*, **55**, 513.
13. Walker, R.A., Senior, P.V., Jones, J.L., Critchley, D.R. and Varley, J.M. (1989) *J. Pathol.*, **158**, 97.
14. Slamon, D.J., Godolphin, W., Jones, L.A. *et al.* (1989) *Science*, **244**, 707.
15. Walker, R.A., Gullick, W.J. and Varley, J.M. (1989) *Br. J. Cancer*, **60**, 426.
16. Seeger, R.C., Brodeur, G.M., Sather, H., Dalton, A., Siegel, S.E., Wong, K.Y. and Hammond, D. (1985) *New Engl. J. Med.*, **313**, 1111.
17. Watson, J.V., Stewart, J., Evan, G., Ritson, A. and Sikora, K. (1986) *Br. J. Cancer*, **53**, 331.
18. Klein, G. and Klein, E. (1986) *Cancer Res.*, **46**, 3211.
19. Bos, J.L. (1989) *Cancer Res.*, **49**, 4682.
20. Blennerhassett, G.T., Furth, M.E., Anderson, A. *et al.* (1988) *Leukemia*, **2**, 648.
21. Grossman, A., Scheer, R.T., Arlin, Z., *et al.* (1989) *Am. J. Hum. Genet.*, **45**, 729.

# 5
# DIAGNOSTIC AND PROGNOSTIC APPLICATIONS OF TUMOR SUPPRESSOR GENES

Less information is available on the practical uses of tumor suppressor genes compared with the oncogenes, primarily reflecting their more recent identification. However, for some of those diseases in which abnormalities in a suppressor gene have been demonstrated, their recognition has had a major effect on patient management. Three diseases in particular have benefited from advances in our knowledge – retinoblastoma, FAP, and most recently NF1.

## 5.1 Retinoblastoma

Retinoblastoma was the first of the inherited cancers in which 'at-risk' individuals could be identified. Sixty per cent of those affected have the unilateral sporadic form of the disease which is non-heritable, and in these individuals the mutation in both copies of the gene can be detected in tumor material but not in somatic tissue. The remainder have a heritable predisposition to the tumors. In approximately 10% of these individuals, the predisposing germ-line mutation has been passed on from a parent. A *de-novo* germinal mutation has occurred in the remainder [1]. As the predisposition is inherited as a dominant trait, children of parents with the heritable form of retinoblastoma are at 50% risk of developing the disease. As the disease is not fully penetrant, a few of the children of unaffected members of families with retinoblastoma are also at risk of subsequently developing tumors.

Both morbidity and mortality can be reduced if diagnosis is made early, so children in families with retinoblastoma are examined frequently. This examination involves ophthalmological investigations, usually under general anesthesia, every 3 months during the first few years of life [2]. Clearly, a predictive test able to differentiate between those at high and low risk could reduce or even eliminate unnecessary examination of 50% of children.

In recent years, detection of individuals at risk from the disease has been made by cytogenetic analysis to detect an obvious deletion encompassing 13q14, by family linkage analysis using polymorphic markers, by detection of a deletion using Southern blotting to estimate gene dosage, or by detection of a rearrangement in the gene which occurs because of the deletion.

Gene carriers were initially identified by linkage analysis with polymorphic markers close to the *RB1* (retinoblastoma 1) locus [3] or with other anonymous probes such as H3-8 [4] which have been shown to be deleted in a number of retinoblastomas. Once the *RB1* gene itself had been cloned, RFLPs detectable within the gene were used. A number of probes have been identified, including those which recognize alterations in restriction enzyme sequences as described in Section 3.1.5, and also one which reflects variation in the number of repeats of a 50 bp sequence (termed variable number of tandem repeats – VNTRs) within the *RB1* gene. This latter probe is particularly informative as there are at least eight alleles in the population. The advantage of using probes which recognize intragenic RFLPs is that they have a low error rate because the chance of recombination between the RFLP and the mutation in the gene is low. It has been possible to use these RFLPs for presymptomatic diagnosis to identify children at high risk of developing retinoblastoma and to identify asymptomatic carriers [5].

The limitation of this type of analysis is that affected family members other than the index case are required for any diagnostic information to be obtained. As three-quarters of heritable cases are the result of a new mutation in the germ cells of the parents, the affected child is frequently the first known case in a family, making linkage analysis impossible. In 3–5% of cases the deletion in affected children can be detected cytogenetically, but the remainder have a sub-microscopic deletion. An alternative method of diagnosis is therefore required. Characterization of the gene and surrounding regions of DNA have made it possible to detect the defect directly in DNA extracted from somatic tissues such as peripheral blood lymphocytes. This technique still requires that the mutation is major, encompassing hundreds of base pairs and is unable to detect point mutations or small deletions.

Initial analysis was performed with the genomic DNA clone H3-8. DNA from the somatic tissues of affected individuals with hereditary retinoblastoma showed a reduction in the intensity of bands detected by the probe as compared with using a DNA sequence from outside the *RB1* region as a hybridization standard. These findings were related to a heterozygous deletion encompassing the *RB1* gene which could not be detected at the microscopic level. In several familial cases, the deletion was shown to be inherited from an affected parent. Approximately 50% of the deletions detected in this way extend as far as the esterase D locus. Those not encompassing this gene were undetectable cytogenetically and therefore range in size from a few up to several hundred kilobases. This technique provided a direct diagnosis in 20% of patients with bilateral disease [4].

Linkage studies using intragenic RFLPs, have provided evidence for major deletions within the *RB1* gene because some affected individuals have only a single *RB1* allele. The inference here is that the mutation in these individuals is a deletion of at least part of the *RB1* gene encompassing the site of the RFLP [5].

cDNA probes covering the *RB1* gene have also been used to detect deletions which give rise to abnormal restriction fragments on Southern blots. These can be detected in the heterozygous form in the DNA isolated from peripheral blood lymphocytes [6]. Tumors from individuals with a constitutional deletion have been shown to be homozygous for the aberrant bands, confirming Knudson's two-hit hypothesis (see Chapter 2).

Other mutations present in the *RB1* gene remain too small to be detected by these means and will require alternative methods for their detection. Where direct detection of the mutation is possible, however, it can differentiate between *de-novo* germ-line mutations and transmission of a mutant gene in asymptomatic carriers. It also provides an alternative method of prenatal diagnosis when linkage analysis is not possible.

### 5.1.1 Alterations in the RB1 gene in other tumors

Patients with the familial form of retinoblastoma frequently develop second tumors such as osteosarcomas after their primary disease has been treated. Structural changes in the *RB1* gene have also been found in these tumors and these have led to the identification of *RB1* mutations in other tumors not associated with retinoblastoma. These include SCLCs, breast cancers, bladder tumors and soft tissue tumors. The results suggest that *RB1* may play a role in malignant transformation or progression in non-hereditary cancers. Deletions in 17% of breast cancers have been detected and although there was no correlation with prognosis, there was a significant correlation with advanced disease [7]. In lung tumors, frequent abnormalities in the *RB1* gene have been seen particularly in SCLC. These changes included absence or trace levels of mRNA in 77% of SCLCs and no *RB1* protein in 100% of cases. In a second study, 31 out of 32 cases of SCLC had a mutation in the *RB1* gene resulting in a complete lack of protein expression. These results suggest a significant role for this gene in SCLC. Evidence for homologous deletions in *RB1* in patients following radiotherapy indicates that the gene may also be a site of mutation following radiation treatment. Further analysis of *RB1* in tumors will hopefully clarify its exact role in tumorigenesis.

## 5.2 Familial adenomatous polyposis

The mode of inheritance of FAP is similar to retinoblastoma and the requirements for presymptomatic testing to prevent unnecessary screening are essentially the same. There are two differences from retinoblastoma. First, the disease is fully penetrant so there are no asymptomatic carriers. Secondly, the *APC* gene has not yet been cloned, so DNA-based diagnosis currently depends solely on linkage analysis.

In this disorder, 50% of the children of an affected individual develop adenomatous polyps. If the polyps are left untreated they will progress to adenocarcinomas in 100% of individuals by the third or fourth decade of life. In addition to polyps in the colon, both gastric and duodenal polyps are seen and there is also an increased risk of periampullary cancer [8]. A related syndrome, originally described by Gardner and named after him, is associated with adenomatous polyps, multiple osteomas, epidermoid cysts and desmoid tumors in a proportion of affected individuals. Gardner's Syndrome and FAP are now believed to be allelic so the diagnostic methods described in this section are appropriate for both.

'At-risk' individuals are offered sigmoidoscopy from about 14 years of age, ideally on an annual basis. This close surveillance should therefore identify early evidence of malignant change before a cancer has had time to develop or metastasize. Patients are then treated primarily by colectomy and ileorectal anastomosis. It does, however, mean that 50% of individuals are screened unnecessarily using a relatively invasive technique. An alternative method of identifying 'at-risk' individuals would therefore be of considerable value both to reduce unpleasant screening procedures and to reduce the costs of unnecessary testing. A number of probes which recognize RFLPs closely linked to the *APC* locus on chromosome 5 have been used in family linkage studies to identify individuals at low risk of developing FAP. In these individuals screening can be reduced or eliminated. Those at high risk can subsequently be followed more closely.

The first marker to show linkage to the *APC* gene – C11p11 – was mapped to 5q21 by *in-situ* hybridization. Unfortunately, its use is limited, as the probe is relatively uninformative; only 20% of individuals are heterozygous [9]. A more informative marker is π227 which recognizes four different polymorphisms, including one in which three different alleles can be detected. This probe is also the furthest from the *APC* gene and carries the highest risk of recombination between it and the gene. Informative individuals have to be given a risk based on an estimated recombination rate of 10% [10]. In the last 2 years several probes closer to the *APC* gene have been identified and at least one of these (YN5.48) has been shown to be located on the distal side of the gene whereas the others are found on the proximal side [11] (*Figure 5.1*). The accuracy of diagnosis in families informative for two of these probes, one on either side of the gene, is greater than 95%. An example of how these probes can be used for presymptomatic diagnosis is shown in *Figure 5.2*. In this pedigree the family are informative with probe π227 and the disease is associated with allele 2. Two of the children (individuals III-1 and III-3) have inherited the low-risk allele (allele 1) from their affected mother and are therefore at only 10% risk (based on the error for this probe) of being affected. In contrast, the second and fourth children have inherited the high-risk allele and are therefore at 90% risk of developing the disease.

A phenotypic marker showing the presence or absence of congenital hypertrophy of the retinal pigment epithelium (CHRPE) is also of diagnostic

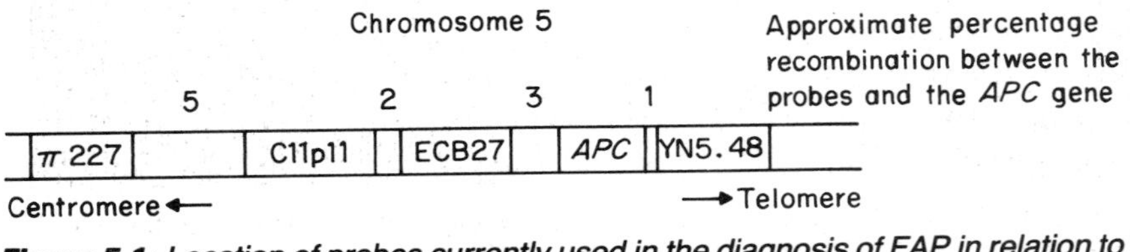

**Figure 5.1:** *Location of probes currently used in the diagnosis of FAP in relation to the* APC *gene.*

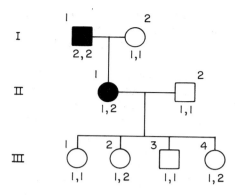

**Figure 5.2:** Pedigree of a family with FAP which is informative with probe π227.

significance (*Figure 5.3*). These lesions are asymptomatic and have been detected in over 80% of those carrying the defective *APC* gene. A combination of the DNA results plus the presence or absence of CHRPE can be used to increase the accuracy of diagnosis [12].

The use of linked probes along with the presence or absence of CHRPE is beginning to have a significant effect on how patients with this disease are monitored. 'At-risk' individuals who have inherited a low-risk allele can either be screened less frequently or not at all, although the latter is currently not recommended as the use of these probes is still in its infancy; world-wide, the number of families tested to date probably constitutes hundreds rather than

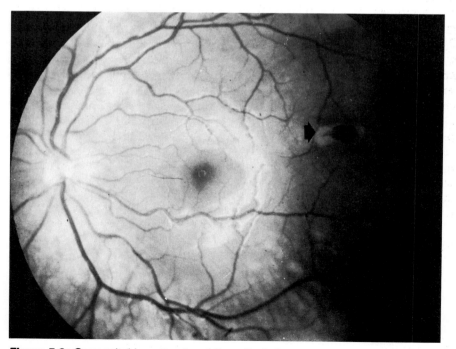

**Figure 5.3:** *Congenital hypertrophy of the retinal pigment epithelium (arrowed). Figure courtesy of Dr J. Gibson, Department of Ophthalmology, East Birmingham Hospital, UK.*

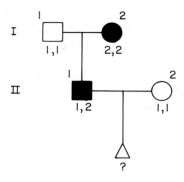

**Figure 5.4:** *Pedigree of a family with FAP, informative with probe YN5.48, who requested prenatal diagnosis.*

thousands. In addition, although there is no evidence of heterogeneity to date, the presence of a second locus cannot yet be completely ruled out.

The other use of linked markers is in prenatal diagnosis. Although the accuracy of such a test is only around 90–95%, this may allow parents to make a decision as to whether a pregnancy should continue. It remains to be determined whether the uptake of this test will be high because there is the possibility of treatment. To date, very few prenatal diagnoses have been carried out for FAP; an example is shown in *Figure 5.4*. This family is informative for YN5.48, the disease segregating with allele 2. DNA was extracted from a chorionic villus biopsy and the fetus was shown to have inherited the low-risk allele from the affected father. The pregnancy could therefore be continued.

A disadvantage with the use of linked probes, apart from the possibility of recombination events, is that DNA from affected family members has to be available for testing for the analysis to have a reasonable chance of success. This is a particular problem in FAP where, until recently, affected individuals frequently died in their thirties. There are many families such as are shown in *Figure 5.5*, in whom linkage studies cannot be used because material is not available from key individuals. This limits the use of these probes in some families. However, methods are becoming available whereby DNA can be extracted from fixed pathology specimens from key individuals who have died. Such DNA is not always of sufficiently high quality for RFLP analysis by Southern blotting, but can often be used in the PCR which is more tolerant of partially degraded DNA. Depending on the size of the PCR reaction product,

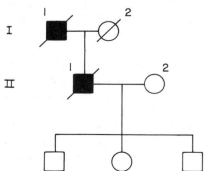

**Figure 5.5:** *Typical pedigree of a FAP family where analysis using linked probes is impossible because key individuals are dead.*

DNA averaging a few kilobases in length can often be used. A polymorphism depending on the presence or absence of a 4 bp deletion has been detected in the C11p11 locus. This can be scored by PCR and may be of value for analyzing DNA from pathology specimens.

Now that markers have been identified on both sides of the gene, the area in which the *APC* gene must lie has been narrowed down and it is therefore only a matter of time before it is finally cloned. Patients can then be assessed directly for evidence of mutations, as is possible now for *RB1* and as will soon be possible for NF1 (see Section 5.3). At the present time, the knowledge that an individual is at low risk of developing cancer can significantly reduce the anxiety for that person.

Identification of this putative suppressor gene in inherited colorectal cancer is also likely to provide valuable information about sporadic colorectal cancer (see Chapter 2), which remains one of the most significant causes of death from cancer in the western world. The region of chromosome 5 containing the *APC* gene has been found to be deleted in 20–50% of sporadic cancers and 30% of polyps, as determined by loss of heterozygosity for chromosome 5q markers [13]. The finding of allele loss in this region in polyps from non-polyposis patients is consistent with the idea that allele loss may be important in colorectal tumorigenesis and may eventually have prognostic significance. Cloning the *APC* gene will also help to clarify further its role in sporadic colorectal cancers.

## 5.3 Neurofibromatosis 1

NF1 is one of the most common autosomal dominant disorders, occurring at a frequency of about 1 in 3000. The spontaneous mutation rate is high and 30–50% of cases are new mutations.

The penetrance of NF1 is extremely high if affected individuals are examined carefully. The diagnostic criteria include at least two of the following: (a) six or more *café au lait* macules; (b) two or more neurofibromas of any type or one plexiform neurofibroma; (c) freckling in the axillary or inguinal regions; (d) optic glioma; (e) two or more Lisch nodules (iris hamartomas); (f) a distinctive bony lesion such as sphenoid dysplasia or thinning of long bone cortex; and (g) a first-degree relative with NF1. As well as optic gliomas, other malignancies, mainly neurofibrosarcomas, can occur [14]. These criteria can be used reliably to diagnose the disease in adults. However, as there is an age-dependent penetrance of these features, it is more difficult to use them to diagnose the disease in children. There is also considerable variation in the expression of the disease, not only between families but also between individuals in the same family. This indicates that the variation in the severity of the disease is not simply due to genetic heterogeneity.

DNA-based testing is therefore of use for presymptomatic testing of children, confirming a diagnosis where only minimal expression of the disease is present, and for prenatal diagnosis if required. The field of NF1 research has moved rapidly in the last few years: in 1987 the disease was mapped to chromosome 17, by 1989 several informative markers were identified flanking the gene, and in 1990 the *NF1* gene itself was cloned.

Initial linkage studies with 31 polymorphic probes linked to the *NF1* gene were performed in 142 families containing 700 individuals [15]. The closest markers on the distal and proximal sides of the gene showed 9% and 4% recombination respectively. This meant that it was feasible to use the markers for presymptomatic and prenatal diagnoses. There was no evidence in this or subsequent studies that the disease was not linked to markers on chromosome 17. This suggests that the disease is genetically homogeneous and that the variability in its clinical expression cannot be explained by mutations in two different genes. The problem with using probes in prenatal diagnosis is the variation in expression of the disease within families. The linked probes can be used to predict high or low risk, but are of no use in predicting the severity of the disease. This may contribute to difficulties in counselling families with NF1 and using the results from linkage studies for prenatal diagnosis. In addition, because of the high new mutation rate, many pedigrees contain only one individual with NF1 which means that analysis by linkage is impossible.

The recent cloning of the *NF1* gene should enable a direct diagnosis to be made, particularly if most of the mutations fall within a limited region of the gene. Two groups of patients with NF1 have been described with translocations which disrupt the gene sequence, one patient has a 500 bp insertion close to or within the gene and three out of 54 patients have germ-line mutations within the region. These mutations have all been instrumental in helping to clone or characterize the gene. In addition, an examination of approximately 10% of the gene in 72 individuals has revealed six mutations spread over four exons [16].

Further information about the gene itself may also correlate the nature of the mutation with the severity of the disease. This may make counselling easier and make a decision on prenatal diagnosis simpler for the patient.

## 5.4 Other tumor suppressor genes

At the present time other tumor suppressor genes have not been used diagnostically. This is likely to change shortly for Wilms tumor with the cloning of the gene. However, families with a heritable predisposition to the disease can only be counselled once it is clear which of the several genes is involved (see Section 2.2.1). Linkage of NF2 to a marker on chromosome 22 is likely to make prenatal and presymptomatic diagnosis of this condition possible. Like the diseases mentioned in the preceding sections, this condition is also inherited in a dominant manner. As NF2 is difficult to detect until symptoms appear, prognostic markers would be particularly useful, both for counselling patients and for monitoring early development of tumors. Similarly, linkage studies of families with multiple endocrine neoplasia (MEN) type-1, mapped to chromosome 11, and MEN type-2 mapped to chromosome 10, are likely to aid counselling of these conditions. Deletion of the short arm of chromosome 3 is a consistent finding in lung cancers, particularly SCLCs where up to 93% of cases are deleted. By analogy with other studies on allele loss, it has been postulated that a 3p deletion is associated with loss of a tumor suppressor gene. Although it has not yet been used diagnostically, the frequency of this finding suggests that a gene on 3p plays an important part in lung cancers and may find a direct application in the future.

Finally, evidence of allele loss in tumors such as breast and ovarian cancers suggests candidate regions in which to begin the search for markers for use in linkage analysis of families with the heritable form of these diseases. Recently, germ-line mutations of the *p53* gene were detected in each of five families studied who suffered from the rare dominantly inherited Li–Fraumeni Syndrome characterized by the presence of diverse tumors, especially breast cancers. The ability to detect mutations in carriers will be a tool for screening members of these families and so detecting the disease presymptomatically. It remains to be seen what the frequency of germ-line p53 mutations is in other cancer patients [17].

## References

1. Vogel, F. (1979) *Hum. Genet.*, **52**, 1.
2. Reese, A.B. (1976) in *Tumours of the eye*, 3rd edn. Harper and Row, Hagerstown, p. 102.
3. Cavenee, W.K., Murphree, A.L., Shull, M.M., Benedict, W.F., Sparkes, R.S., Kock, E. and Nordenskjold, M. (1986) *New Engl. J. Med.*, **314**, 1201.
4. Horsthemke, B., Greger, V., Barnert, H.J., Hopping, W. and Passarge, E. (1987) *Hum. Genet.*, **76**, 257.
5. Wiggs, J., Nordenskjold, M., Yandell, D. *et al.* (1988) *New Engl. J. Med.*, **318**, 151.
6. Janson, M., Kock, E., and Nordenskjold, M. (1990) *Hum. Genet.*, **85**, 21.
7. Varley, J.M., Brammar, W.J. and Walker, R.A. (1989) *Hormone Res.*, **32**, Suppl. 1, 250.
8. Bulow, S. (1987) *Dan. Med. Bull.*, **34**, 1.
9. Bodmer, W.F., Bailey, C.J., Bodmer, J. *et al.* (1987) *Nature*, **328**, 614.
10. Meera Khan, P., Tops, C.M.J., van der Broek, M. *et al.* (1988) *Hum. Genet.*, **79**, 183.
11. Tops, C.M.J., Griffieon, G., Vasen, H.F.A. *et al.* (1989) *Lancet*, **ii**, 361.
12. Houlsten, R., Slack, J. and Murday, V. (1990) *Lancet*, **i**, 484.
13. Fearon, E.R. and Vogelstein, B. (1990) *Cell*, **61**, 759.
14. Collins, F.S., Ponder, B.A.J., Sezinger, B.R. and Epstein, C.J. (1989) *Am. J. Hum. Genet.*, **44**, 1.
15. Goldgar, D.E., Green, P., Parry, D.M. and Mulvihill, J.J. (1989) *Am. J. Hum. Genet.*, **44**, 6.
16. Cawthorn, R.M., Weiss, R., Xu, G. and Viskochil, D. (1990) *Cell*, **62**, 193.
17. Malkin, D., Li, F.P., Strong, L.C., *et al.* (1990) *Science*, **250**, 1233.

# 6

# THERAPEUTIC APPLICATIONS OF ONCOGENES AND THEIR PRODUCTS

Current non-surgical approaches to the treatment of cancer suffer from the major limitation that they are not specific for malignant cells. While chemotherapy significantly improves survival rates in certain tumors, such as ALL and testicular cancer, for most 'solid tumors', which comprise the majority of the cancer incidence and mortality statistics (lung, breast, gastric, colon, ovarian), survival figures have hardly improved over 30 years. In earlier chapters we presented compelling evidence for the importance of oncogenes in the etiology of many human tumors (see also [1] for review). These genes and their encoded proteins are therefore potential targets for attack by specific therapeutic agents. In this chapter we will discuss whether this expectation has been, or is near to being, realized.

Potential targets for therapy include the oncogenes themselves, their RNA transcripts, and their protein products. Initially the expectation was that therapy directed against oncogenes or their products would be more specific to cancer and less harmful to normal tissues of the body. Since, in most cases, oncogene products have proved to be ubiquitous, specific inactivation of oncogenes would have wide-ranging effects. An example of this is the *SRC*-related protein kinases. These were among the first oncogene products to be recognized and specific inhibitors of these kinases seemed logical candidates for anticancer drugs. It is now known that the kinases carry out numerous functions essential to cell survival. Generalized interference with tyrosine phosphorylation would, therefore, have as low a therapeutic index as traditional anticancer drugs. In addition, it is the lack of tyrosine substrate at the end of the cytoplasmic tails of kinase receptors that is responsible for their failure to autoregulate. The tyrosine kinase portions of these oncogene products seem to differ only slightly from their normal proto-oncogene counterparts. Thus, truly specific anti-*ONC* protein inhibitors may be difficult to realize in practice [2].

Several approaches to the therapeutic uses of oncogenes are worth considering.

(a) Antibodies can be used against growth factors and other factors associated with the transformed phenotype, such as enzymes or proto-oncogene products like *RAS* p21. This includes the use of antibodies to focus toxic agents or cells of the immune system on cancer cells.

(b) Oncogenic nucleic acid sequences could be targeted by antisense oligo-nucleotides of DNA or RNA, or by nucleotide antimetabolites such as dideoxy- or methylphosphonate-modified nucleotides.

(c) A mutated activated oncogene might be directly replaced by its non-mutated normal counterpart.

## 6.1 Role of antibodies

### 6.1.1 Use of antibodies as carriers of cytotoxic agents

The idea of targeting drugs to cancer cells using antibodies as carriers is not a new concept: it was proposed early in this century by Paul Ehrlich. However, it is only in the last 20 years that this approach has begun to be tested experimentally and a major impetus to its evaluation was the development of mono-clonal antibodies by Kohler and Milstein in the mid 1970s [3]. As they are derived from the clonal expansion of a single antibody-producing cell, monoclonal antibodies are homogeneous and react with only a single antigenic determinant. The production of such antibodies was clearly a major advance over the polyclonal antisera available previously which contained mixtures of antibodies of varying specificities. In the clinical as well as the experimental setting, this lack of definition made polyclonal antisera less useful for purposes where high specificity was required.

The three basic components necessary for a targeting system are, (a) a target present either exclusively on the tumor cell or at least expressed in greater amount on tumor compared to normal tissue, (b) a carrier or delivery system, and (c) a toxic agent or set of molecules which will cause damage to the tumor after they have been directed there. The objective with this form of targeted therapy (site-specific delivery of drugs or toxins) is to deliver the toxic agent to its site of action on or near the tumor cells, thereby reducing toxicity to normal cells and increasing the therapeutic index of the agent.

Ideally, the target would be present on the tumor and not on any normal cells or tissues. Unfortunately, despite extensive investigation, the existence of tumor-specific antigens remains unproven for the majority of human tumors (but see also Section 6.5.1) and most antibody-mediated targeting has therefore been directed at tumor-associated antigens, many of which are differentiation antigens such as carcino-embryonic antigen, or antigens present on particular cell types such as the melanoma-associated antigens. A variety of other cancer markers have also been tried. Even if no truly tumor-specific targets are available, products of oncogenes that are qualitatively different from normal host products could serve to increase the therapeutic index.

Although a wide variety of carrier systems for the delivery of therapeutic agents to target cell populations have been proposed, the theoretical prerequisites of each should be similar. That is, the carrier should be specific for the target site, it should be able to be linked to the toxic agent without excessive loss of specificity or reactivity and without loss of activity of the agent, and it should remain as a complex until delivery to the target. Additionally, protection of the therapeutic agent from the host's natural defense mechanisms would be desirable, thereby preventing premature inactivation of the conjugate of carrier and toxic agent.

Of all the carrier systems postulated, antibodies have shown the greatest potential and have been the most intensively investigated to date. The use of antibodies to target 'warheads' such as radioisotopes, drugs or toxins has great theoretical appeal because of the unique specificity of the antibody for the target antigen (see *Figure 6.1*). Monoclonal antibodies linked to radioisotopes have been used in diagnostic radioimmunolocalization studies to visualize tumor sites in patients after gamma-camera scanning, and also in studies aimed at therapeutic benefit (see *Figures 6.2* and *6.3*). Toxins linked to monoclonal antibodies have great cytotoxic potency. There is much interest in their use for therapy and for bone marrow purging, for example, removing T cells from bone marrow before allogeneic bone marrow transplantation. They have also proved valuable for treating steroid-resistant graft-versus-host disease. A

Tumor

Normal

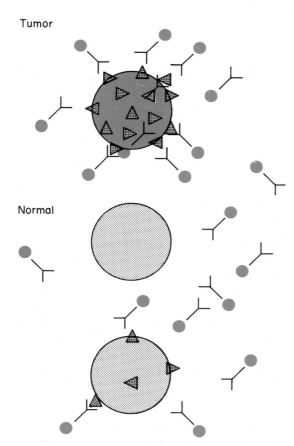

**Figure 6.1**: *Principles of immunotargeting using anti-bodies. Antibodies (●‹) labeled with radioisotope, toxin or chemotherapeutic drug; and membrane-expressed target antigen (▲). Since there is more of the target on the tumor than on the normal cells, there will be a greater accumulation of labeled antibody at the tumor cell. This can be of value in diagnosis and/or therapy.*

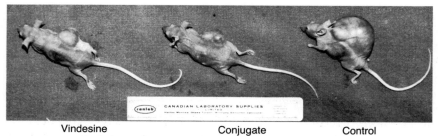

Vindesine                    Conjugate                    Control

**Figure 6.2:** *Representative nude mice from three experimental groups at day 42. On day 0 the nude mice were injected subcutaneously with a human colonic cancer cell line (LS174T) which expresses the target antigen, carcino-embryonic antigen. The treatments the animals received were: control – saline only; vindesine – the chemotherapeutic drug vindesine; and conjugate – an immunoconjugate of a monoclonal antibody to carcino-embryonic antigen to which vindesine molecules had been chemically linked.*

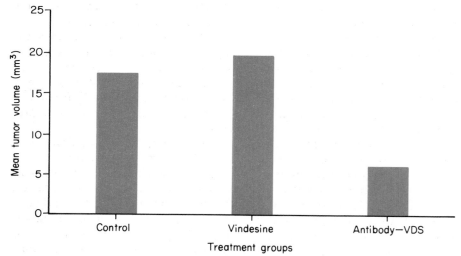

**Figure 6.3:** *Nude mice bearing a human colonic cancer xenograft (WiDr) which expressed carcino-embryonic antigen have been treated with saline (control), vindesine, or an immunoconjugate of vindesine and a monoclonal antibody which recognizes carcino-embryonic antigen (antibody–VDS). The mean tumor volume in the immunoconjugate-treated group is significantly less than in the other two groups.*

detailed discussion of this approach is beyond the scope of this book, but a number of recent reviews [4–8] discuss in depth its potential, advantages and disadvantages. These reviews also describe aspects such as the therapeutic use of monoclonal antibodies linked to radioisotopes, chemotherapeutic drugs or toxins.

One major drawback is, however, worthy of a brief mention. The best monoclonal antibodies for clinical use so far have proved to be of rodent (mainly mouse) origin. In most diagnostic and therapeutic studies involving repeated administrations of these antibodies to patients, human anti-mouse antibodies (HAMA) are produced and these can prevent continued treatment by accelerating clearance of the monoclonal antibody and reducing efficacy. These antibodies can also potentially lead to immune complex deposition and complement activation. One approach to overcoming the development of HAMA has been the construction of murine/human chimeric antibodies by recombinant DNA methodology. As the majority of the host immune response is thought to be directed at the constant C region of an antibody molecule, the production of antibodies with antigen specificity defined by murine variable V regions and C-region domains of human origin could, in theory, reduce the immunogenicity of these molecules. Preliminary trials of these antibodies in patients have confirmed this hypothesis. Readers are referred to recent reviews for the background to the molecular genetics of immunoglobulins [9,10] and genetically engineered antibodies [11,12]. An additional advantage of such an approach is that it is now feasible to change the effector functions of a particular monoclonal antibody by splicing on mouse or human C-region genes of the desired immunoglobulin subclass producing novel effector functions [13,14]. Despite these innovative approaches, recent work has indicated that although chimerization can diminish the anti-antibody response, foreign heavy chain V-region framework regions can be sufficient to lead to a strong anti-variable-region response [15]. A further refinement of this approach has therefore been to replace only the hypervariable or complementarity determining regions (CDRs), rather than the entire V region, of human antibody with rodent CDRs [16,17]. It remains to be seen whether such an approach will overcome one of the major limitations of the therapeutic use of antibodies in patients.

With the discovery of oncogenes in the early 1980s expectations were raised that the oncogenes themselves, or their products, would serve as targets. Many doubted, however, whether this would prove feasible with nuclear oncoproteins. It was difficult to see how the antibody would reach a target in the nucleus. Nevertheless, preliminary evidence indicated that antibodies to some oncogene products, e.g. *MYC*, could be used for radio-immunolocalization studies in, for example, lung cancer (see Section 4.2). Furthermore, those oncogenes coding for products or receptors on the tumor cell surface could provide suitable targets and there are a number of preliminary studies which indicate that such an approach is feasible.

### 6.1.2 Use of antibodies to reverse the malignant phenotype

As discussed in previous chapters, the normal *RAS* protein, p21, differs in several ways from the *RAS* proteins encoded by *RAS* oncogenes. A group of investigators have exploited this difference by microinjecting an antibody against the oncogenic form of p21 into living cells transformed by *RAS* oncogenes [18]. The result was conversion of the transformed cells to a normal phenotype. The antibody did not bind to the normal form of p21 and the revertant cells continued to grow normally. As the microinjected antibody was degraded, the oncogenic p21 was re-expressed and the cells returned to the transformed state. This experiment was important because it demonstrated that an agent capable of inactivating an oncogene product specifically is able to reverse a transformed morphology. However, microinjection of such agents into malignant cells *in vivo* offers little hope as a practical anticancer approach with current biotechnology [2].

### 6.1.3 Antibody-mediated neutralization of other factors associated with the transformed state

Many studies have demonstrated raised levels of proteolytic enzymes associated with malignant tumors *in vivo* and malignant transformation *in vitro*. Activities of collagenases, various cathepsin enzymes, and serine proteases have been shown to be elevated in malignant cells. It has been shown that low concentrations of a monoclonal antibody, selected for its ability to inhibit plasminogen activator, can inhibit the overgrowth and morphological changes associated with Rous sarcoma virus transformation of chick embryo fibroblasts [2]. As in the previous section, this experiment indicated that 'factors' released from malignant cells can be neutralized by monoclonal antibodies.

### 6.1.4 Antibody-mediated targeting of cytotoxic cells

In the mid 1980s it was demonstrated that linking two monoclonal antibodies to make a 'heteroconjugate' (one part recognizing the CD3 component of the T-cell receptor on T cells and the other part recognizing a marker on the tumor cell surface) resulted in activation of T cells at the tumor cell surface with resultant cytotoxicity against the tumor [19]. This is an example of a bispecific antibody, an antibody recognizing two different targets with two antigen-combining sites. Originally, bispecific antibodies were made by chemical cross-linking, but now better methods are available, for example, somatic cell fusions. This involves the fusion of two hybridomas producing monoclonal antibodies, or the fusion of spleen cells, from mice immunized with the target antigen, with a hybridoma already secreting a monoclonal antibody of defined specificity. With these techniques bispecific monoclonal antibodies have been produced which recognize markers on the tumor cell surface and, as well as T cells, cytotoxic drugs and toxins [4] (*Figure 6.4*). Preliminary *in-vitro* results with such antibodies have been very encouraging.

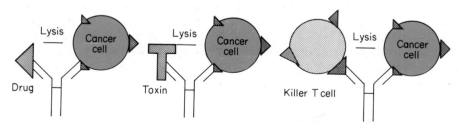

**Figure 6.4:** *Potential of bispecific antibodies. One antigen binding site binds to the target antigen on the tumor cell membrane while the other antigen binding site can be used to focus chemotherapeutic drugs, toxins or cytotoxic cells of the immune system on the cancer cell. Figure courtesy of Dr V. Reddy, Memorial University, Newfoundland, Canada.*

If the target is a membrane-expressed product of an oncogene, there is no reason why this approach should not become of immense value in the destruction of cancer cells.

## 6.2 Potential of growth factors and their receptors as targets for therapy

As indicated earlier, a qualitative difference between growth factors which are produced by oncogenes and their normal counterparts could be sufficient for an improved therapeutic index. An example which fits into this category is the use of antibodies to the *SIS* gene product. However, it should be noted that in some cases anti-autoactive growth factor antibodies have not been able to block continued cell growth. This lack of effect could be the result of intracellular stimulation of growth by autocrine growth factors. Anti-PDGF antibodies, for example, have been shown to inhibit only some *v-sis*-containing cell lines [2].

Monoclonal antibodies reacting with growth-factor receptors may have additional inhibitory effects on tumor cell growth if they block access of growth-stimulating activities to their receptors [20]. A blocking antibody to the receptor for type-I insulin-like growth factor has been used to demonstrate mitogenic effects of insulin-like growth factors on pancreatic carcinoma, neuroblastoma and melanoma cells. This mode of action has also been described for several monoclonal antibodies reacting with the EGFR. However, an antibody which recognizes a protein epitope close to the EGF binding site on the extracellular domain of the EGFR, blocks binding of EGF to both high and low affinity EGFR expressed on the membranes of an *in-vitro* cell line. This effectively inhibits EGF-dependent proliferation of diploid fibroblasts, thus exhibiting an EGF-antagonistic mode of action. TGF-α is a structural homolog of EGF and competes with EGF for binding to the EGFR. A monoclonal antibody has been shown to inhibit binding of TGF-α to the EGFR. In carcinoma cells which express the EGFR, this significantly reduces the growth stimulation elicited by exogenous EGF and TGF-α [20].

Antibodies which bind to the *NEU* oncogene product have been shown to inhibit the growth of cells that express this protein both *in vitro* and *in vivo*. Antibodies against the EGFR also appear to make good immunotoxins. Transferrin receptor expression is generally increased on rapidly growing cells and on some malignant cells in particular. Several research groups have shown that monoclonal antibodies against the transferrin receptor, with attached toxins (ricin, diphtheria), are capable of killing cells over-expressing the transferrin receptor *in vitro*. Such immunotoxins can also inhibit the growth of human tumors growing as xenografts in nude mice [2].

## 6.3 Use of antisense RNA or oligonucleotides

Following the initial discoveries of natural antisense RNAs in prokaryotes, numerous applications of antisense RNA-mediated regulation have been demonstrated in a variety of experimental systems [21,22]. These non-translated mRNAs directly repress gene expression by hybridizing to a target

RNA, rendering it functionally inactive. Specificity of antisense RNA for a particular transcript is conferred by extensive sequence complementarity with the 'sense' or target RNA [22]. Translation of a target mRNA is inhibited following formation of a sense–antisense RNA hybrid. In addition, the duplex molecule may become sensitive to double-strand-specific cellular nucleases. Other effects of antisense RNA may include transcriptional attenuation of the mRNA and also disruption of post-transcriptional processing events [22].

Oncogene DNA and RNA differ in nucleotide sequences from normal proto-oncogene DNA and RNA, and it is therefore theoretically possible to design specific antisense molecules to block translation of oncogene mRNA. For example, by analogy with the microinjection of antibodies against the *RAS* p21 oncogenic product cited earlier, microinjection of antisense DNA sequences might bind to, and block expression of, oncogene DNA. Such 'blocking DNA' could also incorporate an anti-DNA toxin, such as an alkylating agent, to destroy the portion of the chromosome encoding the oncogene specifically. Similarly, an antibody against the oncogenic RNA sequence might bind and prevent that mRNA molecule from being used by ribosomes, or it might inhibit elongation by blocking transfer RNA from binding to the oncogenic messenger anti-codon [2].

Several groups have tried to reverse the transformed phenotype by expressing large amounts of mRNA from the DNA strands complementary to the one coding an aberrant oncogene protein. In the nuclei of the cells the two complementary mRNA strands hybridize to form a double-stranded structure that effectively prevents translation of the mRNA [2] (*Figure 6.5*). Several laboratories are testing retroviruses encoding antisense RNA expressed in a tissue-specific manner by use of appropriate enhancer and other control regions attached to the anticancer genes. To make this approach practical, a better understanding of retroviral tissue tropism mediated by cell surface receptors will be important. It would not be acceptable to infect a cancer patient with a retroviral vector carrying an antisense gene until its efficacy and more importantly its safety have been proved [2].

A novel approach in this same category is the use of oligonucleotides. Antisense oligodeoxynucleotides are one example of a specific therapeutic tool with the potential for ablating oncogenic function. These short (usually <30 bases) single-stranded synthetic DNAs offer the opportunity to modify the expression of genes, including oncogenes, in a sequence-specific manner [23, 24]. Some naturally occurring (e.g. viral) or synthetic [e.g. poly(I)–poly(C)] polynucleotides have been used successfully as antiviral and anti-tumor agents. Their effect may depend on their interferon-inducing properties [2].

Further details of the various classes of compounds currently being evaluated are given in the review by Stein and Cohen [23]. These authors discuss unmodified oligodeoxynucleotides, methylphosphonates, phosphorothioates and antisense oligonucleotides. The advantages and disadvantages of each depend on their efficacy in duplex formation, their nuclease resistance, and the effectiveness of specific gene inhibition.

A number of successful drugs used in cancer chemotherapy, immunological suppression and viral inhibition are analogs of nucleosides. Their use has

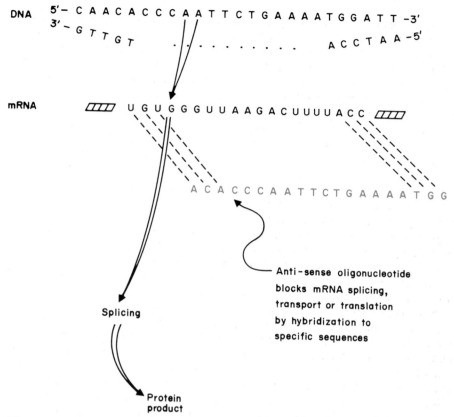

**Figure 6.5:** *Principles of antisense therapeutics. Oligonucleotides or retroviral encoded antisense mRNAs bind to critical control regions (e.g. splice acceptor sites) and prevent the processing, extranuclear transport and translation of selected transcripts. Figure reproduced from [2] with permission from Springer-Verlag.*

previously been limited by cell toxicity owing to *in-vivo* conversion of the nucleoside analogs to nucleotides that become incorporated into cellular DNA, RNA and nucleotide enzymes. However, the use of dideoxynucleosides for treatment of HIV infection has been promising and so far has been associated with low cell toxicity [2].

Clearly this is a promising therapeutic approach to inhibit cancer cell growth. The potential problem of oligonucleotide degradation by nucleases could be overcome using delivery systems based on liposomes or biodegradable polymers, by daily parenteral administration or by synthesis of non-hydrolyzable linkages as in the methylphosphonates. Many years of work and drastic improvements in the potency, stability and targeting of oligodeoxynucleotides are required before these substances can be applied *in vivo*. Antisense oligodeoxynucleotides might be used *in vitro* for some cases of leukemia and lymphoma. Just as antibody immunoconjugates can be used for bone marrow purging (see Section 6.1.1), antisense oligodeoxynucleotides specific for oncogenes might be used selectively to inhibit the growth and survival of residual malignant cells in the bone marrow of patients prior to autologous bone marrow transplantation.

In bone marrow samples obtained from patients with acute leukemia, leukemic cell growth has been reduced selectively, with continued normal hematopoiesis, by the use *in vitro* of specific oligodeoxynucleotides complementary to mRNA of the *MYC* oncogene. This antisense oligodeoxynucleotide inhibits production of the *MYC* protein selectively. In addition, antisense oligodeoxynucleotides complementary to strategic sites in *BCL2* mRNAs have been shown to suppress specifically the proliferation of lymphoma and leukemia cells in culture [23].

## 6.4 Cytokine modulation of oncogenes

In addition to the targets represented by the protein products of oncogenes, there is evidence that the expression of mutant genes is closely linked to aberrant cytokine gene expression. It has been demonstrated that expression of a mutant *RAS* oncogene in at least two different human cell types is associated with significant alterations in the regulation of genes encoding several cytokines, including IL1A, IL1B, CSF2, CSF3 and IL6 [25]. Further elucidation of the mechanism by which *RAS* mutations result in dysregulation of cytokine gene expression should lead to a better understanding of the biological effects of these genetic alternatives in cancer cells, and will possibly reveal new ways of manipulating the growth of malignant cells.

## 6.5 Tumor suppressor genes as targets

The therapeutic possibilities of introducing extra copies of the wild-type *p53* and *RB1* genes into the DNA of tumor cells are readily apparent because the loss of normal function of one, or both, of these gene products has proven to be a frequent event in the developmemt of human cancer. In the case of both *RB1* and *p53*, returning the wild-type allele of these genes into a transformed cell, or a cell undergoing transformation in culture, reverses the tumorigenic potential of the cell or prevents transformation occurring [26]. There is now convincing evidence that both *RB1* and *p53* have the ability to reverse the malignant phenotype when wild-type genes and gene products are expressed in transformed cells. In future it may prove possible to provide extra copies of these tumor suppressor genes, or others that may be identified subsequently, prophylactically to all somatic cells, thus reducing the risk of developing cancer.

### 6.5.1 p53 as a target for therapy

The possibility of new therapeutic approaches is also raised by the fact that p53 protein is so commonly mutated, revealing new epitopes, that a tumor-specific p53 antigen has been demonstrated in the majority of human cancers (see also Section 6.1.1). Over the 10 years since it was discovered, *p53* has progressed from being a curiosity involved in SV40 viral transformation to being the site of the most common genetic change in human cancer and has thereby opened up new therapeutic approaches [27]. As well as the possibilities indicated in the previous section, it may also be possible to immunize patients appropriately with p53 protein and to stimulate a cytotoxic T-cell response against their tumors.

## 6.6 Conclusions and future prospects

Much of the work on oncogene therapeutics is in a preliminary or even speculative theoretical stage. There is considerable enthusiasm for the therapeutic potential revealed by the study of oncogenes; however, we must remember that oncogene products are of fundamental importance to normal cell growth and differentiation, and that mutant oncogenes and their products often differ from their normal counterparts only in minor details. In theory this may be sufficient to improve the current therapeutic index, but it is possible that anti-oncogene therapies may prove as, or more, toxic than the therapeutic modalities currently available.

In addition, with few exceptions, the technical means available to achieve these therapeutic possibilities range from the primitive and experimental to the currently impossible, making practical realization of many of these treatments a good number of years in the future [2].

## References

1. Bishop, J.M. (1987) *Science,* **235,** 305.
2. Buick, K.B., Liu, E.T. and Larrick, J.W. (1988) in *Oncogenes: an Introduction to the Concept of Cancer Genes.* Springer-Verlag, New York, p. 262.
3. Kohler, G. and Milstein, C. (1975) *Nature,* **256,** 495.
4. Ford, C.H.J. and Casson, A.G. (1986) *Cancer Chemotherapy Pharmacol.,* **17,** 197.
5. Ghose, T., Blair, A.H., Uadia, P., Kulkarni, P.N., Goundalalkar, A., Mezel, M. and Ferrone, S. (1985) *Annals N. Y. Acad. Sci.,* **446,** 213.
6. Dilman, R.O. (1989) *Annals Intern. Med.,* **111,** 592.
7. Vitetta, E.S., Fulton, R.J., May, R.D., Till, M. and Uhr, J.W. (1987) *Science,* **238,** 1098.
8. Ford, C.H.J., Richardson, V.J. and Reddy, V.S. (1990) *Ind. J. Pediatr.,* **57,** 29.
9. Taussig, M.J. (1988) *Immunology,* Suppl 1, 7.
10. Williams, A.F. and Barclay, A.N. (1988) *Ann. Rev. Immunol.,* **6,** 381.
11. Morrison, S.L. (1985) *Science,* **329,** 1207.
12. Verhoyen, M. and Reichmann, L. (1988) *BioEssays,* **8,** 74.
13. Neuberger, M.S., Williams, G. and Fox, R.O. (1984) *Nature,* **312,** 604.
14. Bruggemann, M., Williams, G.T., Bindon, C., Clark, M.R., Walker, M.R., Jefferis, R., Waldmann, H. and Neuberger, M.S. (1987) *J. Exp. Med.,* **166,** 1351.
15. Bruggeman, M., Winter, G., Waldman, H. and Neuberger, M. S. (1989) *J. Exp. Med.,* **170,** 2153.
16. Jones, P.T., Dear, P.H., Foote, J., Neuberger, M.S. and Winter, G. (1986) *Nature,* **314,** 268.
17. Riechmann, L., Clark, M., Waldmann, H. and Winter, G. (1988) *Nature,* **332,** 323.
18. Feramisco, J.R., Clark, R., Wong, G., Arnheim, N., Milley, R. and McCormick, F. (1985) *Nature,* **314,** 639.

19. Perez, P., Titus, J.A., Lotze, M.T., Cuttitta, F., Longo, D.L., Groves, E.S., Rabin, H., Durda, P.J. and Segal, D.M. (1986) *J. Immunol.,* **137,** 2069.
20. Rodeck, U., Williams, N., Murthy, U. and Herlyn, M. (1990) *J. Cell. Biochem.,* **44,** 69.
21. Green, P.J., Pines, O. and Inouye, M. (1986) *Ann. Rev. Biochem.,* **55,** 569.
22. Takayama, K.M. and Inouye, M. (1990) *Crit. Rev. Biochem. Mol. Biol.,* **25,** 155.
23. Stein, C.A. and Cohen, J.S. (1988) *Cancer Res.,* **48,** 2659.
24. Reed, J.C., Stein, C., Subasinghe, C., Haldar, S., Croce, C.M., Yum, S. and Cohen, J. (1990) *Cancer Res.,* **50,** 6565.
25. Demetri, G.D., Ernst, T.J., Pratt, E.S. II., Zenzie, B.W., Rheinwald, J.G. and Griffin, J.D. (1990) *J. Clin. Invest.,* **86,** 1261.
26. Levine, A.J. and Momand, J. (1990) *Biochim. Biophys. Acta,* **1032,** 119.
27. Harris, A.L. (1990) *J. Pathol.,* **162,** 5.

# APPENDIX A. CHROMOSOMAL LOCATION OF THE ONCOGENES

| Oncogene | Chromosome | Oncogene | Chromosome |
|----------|------------|----------|------------|
| *ABL* | 9q34 | *KRAS2* | 12p12.1 |
| *ABLL* | 1q24-q25 | *LCO* | 2q14 |
| *AKT1* | 14q32.3 | *LYN* | 8q13-qter |
| *ARAF1* | Xp11.4-p11.2 | *MAS1* | 6q24-q27 |
| *ARAF2* | 7p14-q21 | *MEL* | 19p13.2-cen |
| *BCL2* | 18 | *MET* | 7q31-q32 |
| *CSF1R* | 5q33-q34 | *MOS* | 8q11 or 8q21-q23 |
| *EGFR* | 7p13-p12 | *MYB* | 6q22-q23 |
| *ELK1* | Xp22.1-p11 | *MYC1* | 8q24 |
| *ELK2* | 14q32.3 | *MYCL1* | 1p32 |
| *ERBA2L* | 17q21-q22 | *MYCN* | 2p24 |
| *ERBAL2* | 19 | *NRAS1* | 1p22 and/or 1p13 |
| *ERBAL3* | 5 | *NRASL1* | 9p |
| *ERBB2* | 17q11-q12 | *NRASL2* | 22 |
| *ERG* | 21q22.3 | *PDGFB* | 22q12.3-q13.1 |
| *ETS1* | 11q23.3 | *PIM1* | 6p21 |
| *ETS2* | 21q22.3 | *PVT1* | 8q24 |
| *FES* | 15q25-qter | *RAF1* | 3p25 |
| *FGR* | 1p36.2-p36.1 | *RAF1P1* | 4p16.1 |
| *FOS* | 14q24.3 | *RALA* | 7p22-p15 |
| *GLI* | 12q13 | *REL* | 2p13-cen |
| *HRAS* | 11p15.5 | *ROS1* | 6q21-q22 |
| *HRASP* | Xpter-q26 | *RRAS* | 19 |
| *HRAS2P* | Xp11.4-p11.2 | *SEA* | 11q13 |
| *HSTF1* | 11q13.3 | *SKI* | 1q21.1-q24 |
| *INT1* | 12q13 | *SPI1* | 11p12-p11.2 |
| *INT2* | 11q13 | *SRC* | 20q12-q13 |
| *INT4* | 17q21-q22 | *THRA1* | 17q11-q12 |
| *JUN* | 1p32-p31 | *THRB* | 3p24.1-p22 |
| *KIT* | 4p11-q22 | *YES1* | 18q21.3 |
| *KRAS1P* | 6p12-p11 | *YESP* | 22q11-q12 |

Data taken from *Cytogenetics and Cell Genetics*, Vol. 51: *Human Gene Mapping 10* (1989), with permission from S. Karger AG, Basel.

# APPENDIX B. GLOSSARY

**Allele:** different form of a gene at the same position (locus) on a chromosome.

**Aneuploid:** any chromosome number which is a deviation from the exact multiple of the haploid number.

**Athymic mouse:** see 'Nude' mouse.

**Autosome:** any chromosome other than the sex chromosomes. In humans it refers to chromosomes 1–22.

**cDNA:** complementary DNA – DNA synthesized from mRNA using reverse transcriptase.

**Centromere:** see Chromosome.

**Chromosome:** DNA-containing structure, visible under the microscope in dividing cells. At metaphase of mitosis, a chromosome comprises two identical sister chromatids joined at the centromere (*Figure A1*). In non-dividing cells chromosomes exist as extended single chromatids, not resolvable under the light microscope.

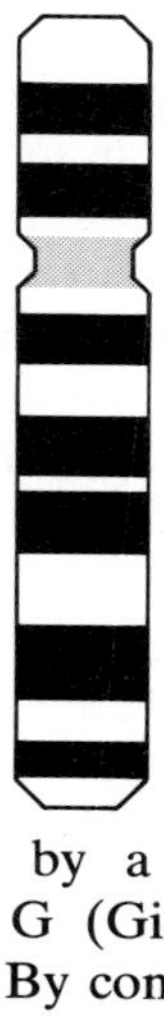

Telomere

Short (p) arm

Centromere

Long (q) arm

Telomere

*Figure A1:* Chromosome structure.

**Chromosome banding:** chromosomes can be stained by a number of techniques. Routinely. they are stained either by G (Giemsa) or R (reverse) banding to give a specific banding pattern. By convention, the bands are numbered separately for the p and q arms, starting at the centromere and working towards the telomere.

**Chromosome walking:** method of moving from a characterized DNA clone known to be near a gene of interest in order to identify that gene. The technique utilizes the ability of the characterized clone to recognize, by homology, further clones containing part of the sequence of the initial clone, but which also contain adjacent DNA sequences along the chromosome.

**Crossing over:** exchange of DNA between homologous chromosomes at meiosis I.

**Diploid:** chromosome number of somatic cells and is twice that of the number found in gametes. In normal humans the diploid number is 46.

**Dominant:** any trait which is expressed in a heterozygote.

**Enzyme-linked immunosorbent assay (ELISA):** assay dependent on the use of an enzyme-labeled antibody to measure antibody or antigen levels. The amount of labeled antibody bound to its target is usually determined by addition of the enzyme's substrate which is degraded to give a colored product which can be measured spectrophotometrically.

**Exon:** region of a gene which contains the coding information.

**Gene:** sequence of nucleotides in the DNA which encodes a single polypeptide. Contains both exons (coding sequences) and introns (non-coding sequences).

Genetic heterogeneity: phenotypically identical forms of a disease caused by mutations at two different loci.

**Genotype:** the genetic make-up of an individual. Used to describe alleles at a specific locus.

**Germ line mutation:** mutation present in the gametes which can be transmitted from parents to offspring.

**Haploid:** chromosome number found in the normal gametes.

**Haplotype:** combination of the genotypes of several closely linked alleles which are inherited together.

**Heat-shock protein:** protein produced by a cell in response to stress.

**Hemizygote:** an individual with one copy of an allele at one particular locus. Arises because only one chromosome (e.g. the X chromosome in males) or part of a chromosome (e.g. where there is a deletion) is present.

**Heterozygote (heterozygous):** individual with two different alleles at the same locus on homologous chromosomes.

**Homozygote (homozygous):** identical alleles at the same locus on homologous chromosomes.

**Hydrophobicity plot:** plot reflecting the distribution of hydrophilic or hydrophobic amino acid residues in a polypeptide. Used to predict those residues likely to be exposed on the surface of a molecule that may contribute to its antigenicity.

**Immortal cell lines:** those capable of continuous growth in tissue culture.

**Immunocompromized mouse:** see 'Nude' mouse

**Interstitial deletion:** deletion of part of a chromosome between two breakpoints.

**Intron:** non-coding sequence, found in the eukaryotic genome, which is spliced out from primary RNA transcript leading to the production of mature mRNA.

**Karyotype:** chromosome make-up of an individual (*Figure A2*).

**Linkage:** inheritance of two or more genes as a single unit because of their close proximity on the chromosome and not because of chance.

**Locus:** chromosomal location defining the position of a gene.

**Meiosis:** reduction cell division resulting in the production of gametes each with a single copy of every chromosome.

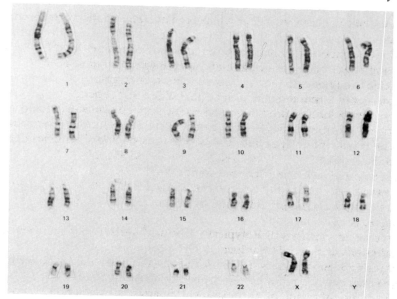

**Figure A2:** *Chromosomal make-up – karyotype – of a normal female. Chromosomes are laid out according to size and banding pattern from chromosomes 1 to 22 plus two X chromosomes.*

**Messenger RNA (mRNA):** product of gene transcription which is subsequently translated into proteins.

**Mitosis:** somatic cell division, whose product is two daughter progeny each with identical copies of every chromosome.

**Monoclonal antibody (hybridoma):** antibody produced by a hybrid cell which is made by fusing a stimulated B cell with a myeloma cell line. The fused cell is clonal and an antibody with a single isotype and a single specificity is produced. Because the myeloma cell is immortal, it can be grown continuously in cell culture providing a continuous supply of identical antibodies.

**Mutation:** a heritable alteration in the DNA sequence.

**'Nude' mouse:** mouse which is immunologically deficient. It can therefore be used to grow tumor cells from humans and other animals without rejection.

**Oligonucleotide:** short sequence of nucleotides. May be synthesized chemically.

**Penetrance:** frequency of phenotypic expression of a gene mutation in affected individuals.

**Peptide:** short amino acid sequence.

**Point mutation:** mutation causing a single base change in the DNA sequence.

**Polyclonal antiserum:** antibody 'cocktail' comprising a range of antibody isotypes recognizing a number of antigenic determinants on a target molecule. Usually isolated from the blood of an immunized animal. The source of the antiserum has a finite lifespan unlike the source of monoclonal antibodies.

**Polymorphism:** two or more different alleles in a population, each of which is present at a frequency greater than that expected by mutational events.

**Promoter:** sequences 5' of a gene which regulate the initiation of transcription.

**Radioimmunoassay:** assay which depends on the use of a radioisotopically labeled antibody to measure either antibody or antigen levels.

**Recessive:** any trait which is expressed only in homozygotes.

**Recombination:** crossing over between loci on homologous chromosomes resulting in a new combination of linked genes.

**Reverse genetics:** the process by which a gene is mapped and eventually cloned without prior knowledge of the biochemical nature of the gene product.

**Reverse transcriptase:** enzyme which produces a DNA sequence from an RNA template.

**Sex chromosomes:** X and Y chromosomes.

**Somatic cell:** any cell in the body except the gametes.

**Sporadic cancer:** non-heritable form of cancer.

**Telomere:** see Chromosome.

**Transcription:** synthesis of RNA from DNA using RNA polymerase.

**Transfection:** method of transfering a DNA sequence into a cell.

**Transgenic mouse:** mouse which has foreign DNA inserted into the germ-line.

**Translation:** synthesis of a protein from a mRNA template.

**Translocation:** transfer of chromosomal regions between non-homologous chromosomes. May be balanced or unbalanced. Usually abbreviated to t followed by the chromosome numbers involved [e.g. t(8;14) which describes the translocation seen in Burkitt's lymphoma].

**Tumor-associated antigen:** antigen found primarily associated with tumors but also expressed on normal and fetal tissues.

**Zinc finger protein:** transcription-regulating protein which has finger-like structures containing a zinc atom.

# INDEX

p53, 16, 30–34, 40, 79, 90
p62, 11, 52, 53, 56, 60, 63, 64, 66
PDGF, 10, 87
Pedigrees, 41–44, 75, 76
Philadelphia chromosome (Ph[1]), 12, 13, 67, 68
*PHL*, 67
Π227, 74, 75
Ploidy (*see* DNA content)
Point mutations, 12, 15, 17, 30, 40, 54, 59, 61, 64, 67
*pol*, 2, 4, 5
Polyclonal antibodies, 45, 82, 97
Polymerase chain reaction (PCR), 39–40, 44, 54, 55, 59, 68, 76
Polyps, 27, 28, 52, 54, 73, 77
Prenatal diagnosis, 76, 78
Prostate cancer, 64
Prostate-specific antigen, 65
Prostatic acid phosphatase, 64
Protein kinases, 11, 12, 67, 81

Radioimmunoassay, 61
Radioimmunolocalization, 57–59, 83
Radioisotopes, 39, 41, 59, 83, 84
*RAF1*, 11
*RAS*, 6, 10–12, 15, 16, 30, 40, 45, 54, 55, 59, 61, 64–67, 82, 85, 90
Recombination, 43, 74
Residual disease, detection of, 68
Restriction enzyme, 24, 38, 39, 41
Retinoblastoma (*RB1*), 21–26, 31, 33, 34, 71–73, 90
Retrovirus, 2–6, 8, 25
Reversal of malignant phenotype, 21, 85
Reverse genetics, 23
Reverse transcriptase, 2, 4, 5
RFLPs, 23, 24, 38, 41, 43, 44, 59, 64, 72, 74, 76
Rhabdomyosarcoma, 27
RNA
  transcripts, 24, 81
  viruses, 2–6
Rous sarcoma virus, 2, 6, 86

Second messengers, 11
Sigmoidoscopy, 74

*SIS*, 10, 15, 87
Site-specific delivery, 82
Somatic cell hybrids, 19–21, 34
Small cell lung cancer (SCLC), 31, 33, 57–59, 62, 73, 78
Southern blotting, 37–39, 40, 41, 76
Sphenoid dysplasia, 77
*SRC*, 4, 10, 81
Stomach (gastric) cancer, 55–57, 81
SV40, 2, 30, 90

Targeting, 57, 59, 82
T cells, 83, 86, 91
Testicular cancer, 30, 64, 81
TGF
  α, 57, 87
  β, 34
Therapeutic index, 82, 91
TNM staging, 59
Toxins, 83, 84, 86
Transcription factors, 11–12, 27
Transferrin, 87
Transgenic mice, 16
Translocation, 6, 8, 12–14, 28, 65–68, 78, 98
Transplantation, 83
Tumor-associated antigen, 52, 82, 98
Tumor-specific antigen, 82
Two-hit hypothesis (*see* Knudson's 'two-hit' hypothesis)

Ulcerative colitis, 52

Variable number of tandem repeats (VNTRs), 72
Vindesine, 84, 89
V-region, 85
*v-sis*, 6, 87

WAGR, 27
Western blotting, 45–46, 59, 61
Wilms tumor, 26–27, 29, 34, 78

Xenografts, 87

YN5.48, 74, 76

Xeroderma pigmentosum, 1